THE ANTIBIOTIC PARADOX

How Miracle Drugs
Are Destroying the Miracle

THE ANTIBIOTIC PARADOX

How Miracle Drugs
Are Destroying the Miracle

Stuart B. Levy, M.D.

PLENUM PRESS • NEW YORK AND LONDON

Library of Congress Cataloging-in-Publication Data

Levy, Stuart B.
    The antibiotic paradox : how miracle drugs are destroying the
  miracle / Stuart B. Levy.
       p.   cm.
    Includes bibliographical references and index.
    ISBN 0-306-44331-7
    1. Drug resistance in microorganisms. 2. Antibiotics.   I. Title.
  QR177.L48   1992
  615'.329--dc20   92-19936
                                                                  CIP

---

10 9 8 7 6 5

ISBN 0-306-44331-7

© 1992 Stuart B. Levy
Plenum Press is a division of Plenum Publishing Corporation
233 Spring Street, New York, N.Y. 10013

Printed in the United States of America

To

Suzanne and Arthur
and all future generations

PREFACE

Antibiotics have been called the single most important therapeutic discovery in the history of medicine. While other medications could compete for this distinction, antibiotics as a class have clearly revolutionized our ability to curb death and disease from infectious microorganisms. An interesting feature of their historic discoveries is that they occurred within the lifetime of many of the population living today.

The ability of antibiotics, such as penicillin, to effect rapid cures for previously fatal infections led to their being touted as "miracle drugs." This claim remains today, having been passed down through several recent generations. While, to some extent, antibiotics have merited this appellation, it paradoxically has caused some dent in their armor. The seemingly endless miracles attributed to these drugs have led to their misuse and overuse. Bacteria responded to the widespread applications of antibiotics by finding ways to become resistant, in other words, insensitive to the killing effects of these powerful drugs.

Thus, antibiotics sow the seeds of their own potential downfall by selecting for rare strains of bacteria that have the ability to resist their activity. To complicate matters further, many of these resistance traits can be transferred or spread from one kind of resistant bacteria to other bacteria, even of different types.

This adverse result of antibiotic use, a phenomenon that I call the "antibiotic paradox," does not mean that antibiotics have failed or that antibiotics cannot still be used. It simply reflects the dual nature of the powerful effects they have and why they should be used prudently. Fortunately, antibiotics remain very effective in the treatment of a vast majority of bacterial infectious diseases. This situation, however, is not secure and is changing continually. In many parts of the world, cost-effective, inexpensive, and safe antibiotics are no longer successful because of the bacterial resistance to them that has developed. Effective treatment is absent in many parts of the world where newer drugs developed to treat resistant bacteria are too expensive to be made available on the limited national budgets of these developing countries. Therefore, the older antibiotics continue to be used despite growing resistance patterns and, in turn, continue to propagate new and often more resistant types of bacteria. Also, the distribution of these drugs is often uneven. In some areas, antibiotics are being over-used, while in other areas, often those needing them the most, they are drastically underused because of a lack of availability. Hence, the general "use" of antibiotics needs improvement in all parts of the world.

The aim of this book is to explain where and when antibiotics are useful and why they are so valuable. On the other side, there are various uses of antibiotics that should be changed and even curtailed. Our goal is not to suggest the removal of antibiotics from the physician's armamentarium but, in fact, to encourage making them even *more* effective by curbing the emergence and spread of resistant forms of infectious bacteria.

This goal of improving antibiotic use must concern all members of society using these drugs, namely: consumers, whether they be humans, animals, or the agriculture industry; prescribers, whether they be physicians, veterinarians, or plant pathologists; and the producers and companies that are making and marketing these drugs. By recognizing the different areas in which antibiotic use can be improved, we can hope to stimulate better distribution and application, increase awareness of the benefits to be reaped, and curb the threat posed by resistance. The worldwide aim is to protect the effectiveness of these precious natural resources.

Stuart B. Levy, M.D.

Boston, Massachusetts

ACKNOWLEDGMENTS

I thank Linda Regan, Victoria Cherney, and Naomi Brier of Plenum Publishing Corporation for their important insights, suggestions, and probing questions, which helped me put these thoughts together and kept me on the path, aware of my audience. Much appreciated were their continued interest and encouragement.

I am particularly grateful to my long-term associate Bonnie Marshall for her immense help during the final stages of this project, including repeated editing of the text and the superb rendition of the concepts into pictures and graphics. I thank Herbert Hächler, another one of those rare scientists with an artist's flair, for his "made-to-order" cartoons that are on target and certainly liven up the text.

I greatly appreciate the help and information received from Anne Vidaver, Thomas Sullivan, Margaret Erwin, Hachiro Shimanuchi, Howard Myers, Charles Bramble, and Neil Pelletier in the preparation of the sections dealing with non-human uses of antibiotics. I thank Cameron Macauley for his help in researching the material for Chapter 1 and Peter Steere for assistance in the pharmaceutical details.

I also thank those who contributed photographs, in particular Angelo dePaola, who also shared the catfish operation with me as well as so many of the interesting details about raising catfish.

I appreciate the hospitality of Mr. Richard Wolfe of the rare books section of the Countway Medical Library, where I was able to gather so much first-hand material dealing with the history of medicine.

Special thanks go to Claire Sherman, Anne Ryan, Kenneth Ratzan, Jay Levy, Stephen Beal, and Patricia Suzman for their helpful comments on the text.

I particularly thank my wife, Cecile, for her loving support throughout this venture, and my laboratory for providing me with the interesting experimental results relating to this subject.

CONTENTS

Chapter 1

FROM TRAGEDY
THE ANTIBIOTIC AGE
IS BORN

"450 DIE AS FLAMES AND PANIC TRAP COCOANUT GROVE CROWD. . ."[1] screamed the headlines of the *Boston Herald* on Sunday morning, November 29, 1942, filling almost the entire top half of the front page (Figure 1.1). The *Boston Sunday Globe* likewise flashed "400 DEAD IN HUB NIGHTCLUB FIRE. HUNDREDS HURT IN PANIC AS THE COCOANUT GROVE BECOMES WILD INFERNO."[2] This was the most devastating fire in the history of Boston and the worst in America since Chicago's Iroquois Theater disaster in 1903 that killed 575 people. The Cocoanut Grove disaster could have been even worse, had not advances in medical treatment in the previous 40 years helped in the survival of many victims.

The fire also occasioned a medical event now regarded as historically momentous as the fire itself—the trial of a new, unique drug available only through government sources. Limited amounts of "penicillin," an unknown substance, were released to quell many of the infections contracted by survivors of the fire. Until

1

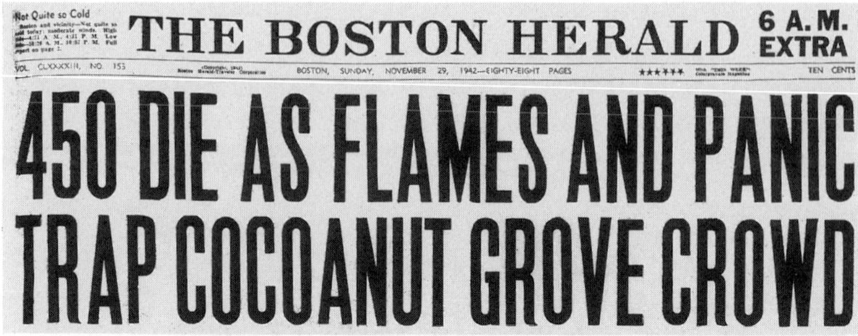

Not Quite so Cold

THE BOSTON HERALD 6 A.M. EXTRA

VOL. CLXXXXIII. NO. 153   BOSTON, SUNDAY, NOVEMBER 29, 1942—EIGHTY-EIGHT PAGES   ★★★★★   TEN CENTS

450 DIE AS FLAMES AND PANIC TRAP COCOANUT GROVE CROWD

Figure 1.1. "The fire that made penicillin famous." It was in treating victims of this Boston fire that penicillin had its first large and publicized clinical trial. The mystery surrounding this "priceless substance" and its acclaimed remarkable powers pushed the United States government and American companies to proceed with its mass production (*The Boston Herald*).[1]

then, the public had little or no conception of this drug's success in treating and preventing life-threatening infections.

The Cocoanut Grove was one of a number of entertainment establishments in Boston, like many in other cities throughout the country, where people went to get away from the agonies and disappointments of World War II that confronted them daily. Over its 15-year history, the club had maintained its reputation as "the" place to be and to be seen. That Saturday night had been no exception.

The club was teeming with its biggest crowd ever. An estimated 800 to 1,000 people crammed its rooms. Servicemen in town for a weekend of relaxation conversed with the locals. Fans from Holy Cross College were there to celebrate after an upset football victory over Boston College. By a certain irony, the Boston College team players were spared the tragedy. Discouraged by their loss, they had gone to bed early, foregoing the evening's planned festivities at the Cocoanut Grove.

The nightclub was located at Piedmont Street and Shawmut Avenue in Boston's South End, adjoining the theater district. Crucial to the chaos that immediately followed the first sign of fire was the single revolving door entrance on Piedmont Street, which led into the main foyer. It was here that hundreds of customers scrambled to get out, only to be crushed and then suffocated in the panic. The nightclub's tenor, Billy Payne, saved ten customers by leading them into the basement icebox and later out to safety. He had been scheduled to open the show with the "Star Spangled Banner" when a screaming, young woman who was afire stopped the show. Some found refuge on the roof, but most people were trapped inside.

The crowd was in full regalia at the time the fire started, a tragic accident ignited by a young barboy with a lighted match. In an interview that night he told a *Boston Globe* reporter, "I was standing in the dining room talking to the bartender. . . . everything seemed to be all right. . . . all of a sudden, a palm tree, one of those phony ones, went up in flames right before our eyes. I never saw anything like it."[3] By the next day this 16-year-old found out that he was the linchpin of the tragedy.

For days, news of the fire filled the front pages of both city newspapers, relegating even the war to secondary status. More prominent were long lists of those injured in the fire, as well as tallies of the dead and headlines like "Where Bodies Can Be Found."[3]

The majority of the more than 400 victims were taken to the two large city hospitals, while the others were distributed among ten smaller ones for treatment. The havoc at these hospitals necessitated sorting the victims, initially into living and dead, and then into those needing limited or more extensive treatment. More than half the victims who arrived were dead or died within five minutes of their arrival. Of the 114 people arriving at the Massachusetts General Hospital, 75 were dead. In all the hospitals, an estimated 200 went directly to the morgue.

Physicians caring for the more than 200 victims who survived the first 24 hours saved more lives than recorded previously for fire victims. They attributed this success to two recent medical therapies. One was an antibacterial, sulfadiazine, a member of the then relatively new class of infectious-disease-killing agents, the sulfonamides, which controlled potentially lethal blood infections caused by the bacterium *Streptococcus*. The other was blood plasma, which was given intravenously to these victims to counteract dehydration caused by fluid loss from the burned surfaces.

Plasma is the fluid part of blood in which the red and white blood cells of the body circulate. Plasma helps maintain a healthy water content in the tissues of the body. The skin is a major protective organ that also maintains balanced body water and temperature. Small amounts of water lost through evaporation through the skin are made up by daily intake of fluids. When the skin is destroyed, as in a severe burn, large losses of water and plasma occur, which can lead to shock and death. In this instance, fluid replacement by mouth is not rapid enough nor sufficient to prevent the potentially fatal consequences.

Almost three-quarters of the burn victims who survived the initial 24 hours sustained large fluid losses through their burns. By giving back plasma, doctors were able to replace lost fluid and body salts, avoiding severe dehydration, shock, and death for an estimated 150 burn victims. At the time of the fire, the technology for separating plasma from blood cells and supplying it for injection into the bloodstream was only four years old. Thus, Cocoanut Grove burn victims were among the first to benefit from this new therapy. A total of 1300 units, taken from 1300 donors, were used during this critical period in the treatment of burn victims.

Yet another new medical treatment, virtually unknown at the time, appeared at one hospital. The Massachusetts General Hospital received a new drug that was made available for use in preventing fatal infections by other bacteria. According to the December 2, 1942, issue of *The Boston Globe*, Merck and Company in Rahway, New Jersey rushed a 32-liter supply of a "priceless" drug to the Massachusetts General Hospital. With police escorts, it made a 7-hour, 368-mile drive through four states in steady rain from its New Jersey production site to the hospital.[4] The drug was penicillin, not in pure form, but actually delivered in the culture liquid in which the drug was produced by a *Penicillium* mold. It combatted *Staphylococcus aureus*, a frequent bacterial contaminant of skin wounds of fire victims.

Once the protective skin is damaged, staphylococci can enter the body, where they circulate and multiply in the bloodstream, leading to high fevers, shock, and death. Prior to the Cocoanut Grove fire, there were no agents readily available to treat this bacterium. Once infections occurred, most patients died. Staphylococci were also the cause of failure of skin grafts, since the microorganisms set up infections on the exposed skin surfaces. The trial use of this new drug presaged its future significance.

Penicillin was described officially as a "medical safeguard against infection." It was still a highly guarded secret and was reserved for military use only. But for victims of this fire, it was released by the government in what became one of its most important clinical trials. The success of skin grafting and treating the severely burned patients was largely attributed to the action of penicillin. This single event has been labelled "crucial" in prompting the United States government to back pharmaceutical houses in their production of penicillin in large amounts.

The enticement of the United States into pursuing penicillin—which has been called a British discovery—followed diplomacy and persistence by the drug's leading developer and protagonist, Howard Florey. Although he did not discover penicillin—that honor goes to a fellow countryman, Alexander Fleming—he and his colleagues are credited with producing it and with demonstrating the drug's success in therapy. Florey, along with Norman Heatley, his colleague and fellow chemist, had made a special trip from England to the United States in the summer of 1941 to expound the wonders of penicillin and to persuade the United States government to back large-scale production. Florey and his team saw this effort as essential for treating casualties of the war abroad and at home, but the financial constraints caused by the war made production impossible for Great Britain. The Cocoanut Grove fire occurred about a year after the visit by these British scientists. Although small amounts of penicillin had been made available and were used successfully in a limited number of patients in the United States, no United States commitment toward production of the drug had been made. During the year since the British visit, other American physicians had received small amounts of the precious new substance and reported "miraculous" results. The glowing reports made the large pharmaceutical houses aware of the new compound's powers. Still, there was hesitation in putting the huge amount of resources needed behind production of a relatively unknown entity. Moreover, giving people penicillin, a natural product of a microorganism, still seemed a questionable idea.

Penicillin's use in treating some of the victims of the Cocoanut Grove tragedy received far more attention than the number of patients treated. Still, very little penicillin was available. Fewer than 100 people in the United States had been treated with it before the fire. It was difficult to purify and its full effects were not known. Drug manufacturers and the United States government demanded proof of its worth and lack of toxicity before mass production could be initiated. The national attention brought to penicillin by the "infamous disaster" did the job. Certainly it was thanks to other medical measures that so many victims lived. But the media focused special attention on the new drug, penicillin. The news accounts provided a widely publicized forum for relating its unknown prior successes, namely accounts of treated patients who were cured of life-threatening infections. Meanwhile, the enthusiasm for producing penicillin reached new heights.

Penicillin earned the accolade "miracle drug" because of its unique and rapid control of infectious bacteria that, before its discovery, had been fully expected to kill the patient. Small amounts of the drug cured blood-borne infections, pneumonias, and open skin wounds. The discovery of sulfonamides in the mid-1930s had revived the quest for what the 19th century German chemist Paul Ehrlich called a "magic bullet," that is, a drug that would kill bacterial invaders without harming the body. Penicillin seemed to be the epitome of the concept. It killed bacteria that the sulfonamides could not affect and produced fewer side effects. It maintained its activity while penetrating dying tissue, a feature that no other drug had demonstrated.

Penicillin clearly symbolized our ability to outwit and control the microbial world. Ironically, the drug itself was not man-made, but a product of molds—natural participants of the microbial environment. For such naturally occurring substances that killed bacteria, the term "antibiotic" was coined.

Amidst the deserved optimism surrounding the successes of penicillin, hovered words of caution. The British bacteriologist Alexander Fleming, who discovered the drug, warned in a 1945 interview by *The New York Times* that misuse of penicillin could lead to the selection and propagation of mutant forms of bacteria resistant to the drug. He had derived such mutant bacteria in the laboratory by growing susceptible bacterial strains in increasingly higher amounts of penicillin, starting with very small amounts of the drug. These mutant bacteria had cell walls that were much less permeable to penicillin, so the drug could not penetrate the bacteria and kill them. These bacteria could resist the levels of penicillin that normally circulated in the blood during treatment with the drug. Fleming, hoping to avoid producing these mutants in patients during therapy, spoke out for complete courses of treatment, since inadequate treatments were more likely to select for, and lead to overgrowth of, these resistant forms.

Fleming predicted that this situation would be worse when the drug became available in an oral form. Then it could be taken easily by patients in their homes without the necessity of intravenous therapy, which required hospitalization. Drug use was monitored in hospitals. On the outside, this would be hard to do. He warned the medical world that

> the greatest possibility of evil in self-medication is the use of too small doses so that instead of clearing up infection, the microbes are educated to resist penicillin and a host of penicillin-fast organisms is bred out which can be passed to other individuals and from them to others until they reach someone who gets a septicemia or a pneumonia which penicillin cannot save.[5]

These early words predicted a phenomenon, namely that resistant bacteria would be selected by misuse of antibiotics and that resistant strains selected in one person, who might remain unaffected, could spread to another. The other person could come down with a form of the disease now insensitive to penicillin. Nevertheless, there was great interest in providing medications that could be given by mouth. Intravenous therapy was not as convenient then as it is today. Hospitals did not have the sterile plastic tubings and disposable needles we have now. Intravenous therapy required reusable materials that had to be sterilized after every use. The availability of oral medications would avoid these cumbersome necessities and make treatments far easier.

When the drug became available orally, it was a major break-through, but as Fleming warned, it was also a sure invitation for misuse. Until the mid-1950s, it was available without a doctor's advice. The drug appeared in over-the-counter preparations and was advertised to the public (Figure 1.2). This free access to penicillin led to its use for diseases not responsive to antibiotics. Moreover, even if there were a bacterial cause, a patient taking less than an optimal dosage would not totally eradicate the infectious agent. Bacteria surviving the incomplete treatment could continue to multiply and among them would be mutants with less suscep-tibility to the antibiotic—like the ones Fleming produced in the laboratory.

But Alexander Fleming's predictions were borne out in a more devastating way than even he surmised. He did not imagine, nor did anyone else at the time, that mutations were not the only way by which bacteria could become resistant. Rare traits already existed in nature that enabled the bacteria, not only to resist the drug, but to actually destroy it. Proteins for destroying penicillin made bacteria much more resistant to penicillin than did the cell wall mutants that Fleming produced in the laboratory. The syn-thesis of these proteins was dictated by genetic material, that is, genes, newly acquired by these bacteria. Penicillin resistance genes, harbored in small numbers of bacteria, were soon found in others, meaning that they could be transferred among the bac-teria. As a result, each new progeny becomes a resistant one and a potential donor of resistance traits to new recipient bacteria.

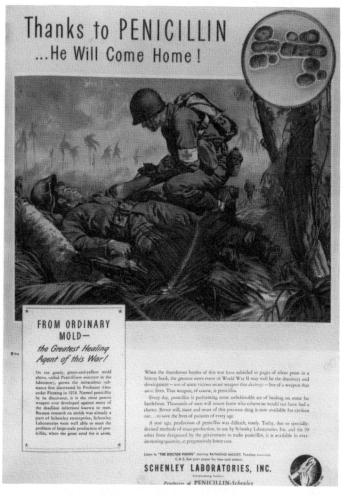

Figure 1.2. When penicillin was first introduced it was not a prescription drug. It was not until the mid-1950s that prescriptions were required. Many companies advertised penicillin to the general public as soon as enough became available. This advertisement appeared in the August 14, 1944 issue of *Life* magazine.

Under optimal growth conditions, one resistant bacterium can reproduce itself in less than an hour. Thus, in a matter of hours, thousands of copies of the original bacterium, and those that received the resistance gene, can emerge.

The rapid appearance of penicillin-resistant staphylococci sobered the euphoria that followed the discovery of penicillin. In London, these penicillin-destroying staphylococci appeared in hospitals where much of the early use of penicillin had taken place. By one account in 1946, just a few years after the introduction of penicillin, 14% of the strains isolated from sick patients were resistant. By the end of that decade, the frequency had jumped to 59% in the same hospital. Initially, and for the ensuing decade, these resistant strains were concentrated in city hospitals. Then, through the 1960s and 1970s they began to surface elsewhere—first in community hospitals and then among strains from people living in those communities.

The success of penicillin encouraged scientists to search for and discover new antibiotics that could treat other bacteria, including penicillin-resistant strains. Chemists developed the means to modify penicillin so that it was not subject to the enzymes that degraded penicillin. As more antibiotics were discovered, from the late 1940s into the 1970s, the problem of resistance seemed little more than an annoyance. Most major human disease agents remained susceptible to many of the common antibiotics or to other new ones. Then, two events in the mid-1970s marked a dramatic change in this complacent mindset. Two different kinds of common infectious bacteria, one which causes ear infections and meningitis in children, and another which causes the venereal disease gonorrhea, emerged with resistance to penicillin. These events occurred in patients in two different parts of the world.

Two infants, 12 and 18 months old, were hospitalized with meningitis in the Naval Hospital in Bethesda, Maryland, one in late 1973 and the other in early 1974. The suspect organism was *Hemophilus influenzae* and the infants were given ampicillin, a penicillin derivative. They died two days later. No one would have expected resistance to this antibiotic since *Hemophilus* bacteria were known to be exceptionally susceptible to ampicillin. In these two patients, however, the *Hemophilus* strains did not respond to the drug. The children, who went to the same day-care center, had picked up strains that were highly resistant, an event that was unexpected after decades of successful ampicillin use. These unique strains had acquired the ability to destroy ampicillin and other related penicillins.

The long-waged war against the ancient scourge, gonorrhea, was presumably over when the early trials with penicillin in the 1940s showed that just a single injection of a small amount of the drug could effectively kill the microorganism. Penicillin could also cure syphilis, another venereal disease often occurring in the same individual. Thus, a single drug could treat two infectious agents potentially present in the same person. But in the mid-1970s, 30 years of success came to a halt. About the same time as *Hemophilus influenzae* appeared with penicillin resistance, so did *Neisseria gonorrhoeae*, the bacteria causing gonorrhea. The resistant strains were also able to destroy the drug. In fact, the enzyme in *N. gonorrhoeae* that destroyed penicillin was the same one found in *H. influenzae*. The identical gene had been picked up by these two different kinds of bacteria. The resistant gonococci were initially discovered in ill servicemen in the Philippines and traced to brothels in Vietnam where penicillin had been given on a regular basis to keep the women "free of disease." Scientists believe that this constant flow of penicillin led to the emergence of rare, never-before-encountered, resistant forms. Since the strains were not contained early enough, they travelled, presumably with infected individuals and with nonsymptomatic human carriers of the bacteria, to the United States and Europe. Today penicillin-resistant gonorrhea strains plague every country of the world.

We can no longer expect that any infection will be cured by the first antibiotic chosen. In some parts of the world, limited supplies of antibiotics mean that *no* available antibiotic is effective. This is a far cry from the situation just twenty years ago. Resistance takes its toll in deaths where newer antibiotics are unavailable or in patients in whom an antibiotic's side effects precludes its use. Patients are suffering and dying from diseases that some predicted forty years ago would be wiped off the face of the earth.

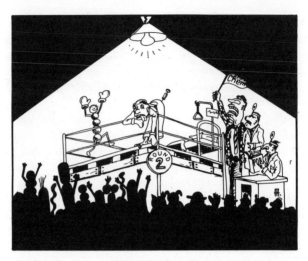

Figure 1.3. The discovery of penicillin led to considerable confidence in winning the fight against bacteria. This dream was short-lived with the emergence of bacterial strains resistant to the drug, first in hospitals and then in the community. While the first round was won by human ingenuity, round two looked like a win for bacteria (Herbert Hächler, University of Zurich, Zurich, Switzerland).

Clearly, the battle we wage with microbes, initially considered won by our enlarging pharmacy of antibiotics, was not an all-out victory for either side (Figure 1.3).

What is the relationship between the use of antibiotics and the emergence of these resistant forms of bacteria? How do these resistances find their bacterial hosts and vice versa? How do we, the consumer or the physician, participate in what appears to be a seesaw experience with bacteria—first a win and then a loss? No matter what we do, the bacteria seem to be able to fight back. These are critical questions at a time when bacteria worldwide are becoming resistant to many different antimicrobial agents. To make matters worse, there are no truly new families of antibiotics that we can expect to be available in the present decade. This means we must make use of the antibiotics that we already have.

Chapter 2

THE DISEASE AND THE CURE

The Microscopic World of Bacteria and Antibiotics

As we go about our everyday activities, we are continually interacting with free-living, single-cell microorganisms invisible to the naked eye. In 1674, a Dutch dry goods merchant, Anton van Leeuwenhoeck, first viewed tiny creatures, "wee animalcules," moving under his hand-sized, homemade microscope. He reported and described his novel findings in letters and drawings, which he sent in 1676 to the Royal Society of London. His discovery opened our eyes and our minds to the existence of living matter that could not normally be seen by the eye. These microscopic beings made up an exotic, previously unimagined world that shared our environment.

But it would take 200 more years before the scientific world would accept bacteria as anything more than interesting creations of nature. That microorganisms could cause illness, the basis of the "germ theory of disease," remained a controversial idea well into the middle of the 19th century. By then, support of the concept was mounting, largely through the observations and tenacious arguments of Louis Pasteur, who was working in Paris. He reported that these bacteria, "microbes," as the French physician Charles Sedillot suggested in 1878, were not spontaneously generated from matter, but were present in the air and from there settled onto exposed living tissue, causing it to decompose. His work and theory were accepted and endorsed formally in a statement by the French Academy of Sciences in 1864. Through his findings and carefully prepared experiments, the French chemist set infectious disease on a totally new path and ultimately completely altered our views of disease. This major revelation occurred only 100 years ago.

With Pasteur's discoveries and interpretations, scientists could begin to understand other events in the environment in a new way. Not only the mystery surrounding the decay of living tissue, but the role of microbes in food production became clear. It was the activity of microscopic beings that caused juices to turn to wine and bread to rise. This understanding paved the way for new breakthroughs in the food industry. More importantly, this discovery of bacteria as active participants in mankind's environment allowed them to be considered as causative agents of human disease.

As the germ theory of disease gained acceptance, scientists discovered that infectious agents were the cause of many well-known illnesses whose treatment had been directed previously at multiple symptoms and organs. There evolved a new recognition that a single microorganism could cause an affliction of many organs of the body. The same disease-causing agent could bring about chills, fever, and also sore throat. For the first time, physicians could link a patient's complaints, formerly described in terms of pains and discomforts, to a microbial cause. Diarrhea was caused by certain toxin-forming bacteria that entered the intestinal tract. Burning on urination occurred because of the irritation of the bladder and urethra created by bacteria growing there. Bacteria could be found and identified in the urine. Cough and difficulty in breathing, along with fever and malaise, could be attributed to a single bacterial cause whose most important effect was on the lung, leading to the disease known as pneumonia.

In 1881, Robert Koch furthered diagnostic and medical knowledge by introducing a solid medium in plates on which to grow and distinguish bacteria. This inventive country physician devised this potato extract, a gelatin and agar mixture, in his home kitchen in Germany. He surmised, and later showed, that a single bacterium would stick to a site on the hardened agar surface where it would multiply to form a colony of hundreds of millions of progeny after overnight incubation (Figure 2.1). Each colony on the artificial medium represented the progeny from a single viable microbe. Bacterial types could be determined in urine, feces, sputum, and other clinical specimens taken from the patient. By diluting and plating specimens on the agar surface and counting the colonies after overnight incubation, he could determine the number of microorganisms present.

Scientists distinguished these colonies by their shapes, texture (smooth or rough borders), size, and color (such as translucent, white, red, or yellow). The progeny of the same type of bacteria formed the same kind of colony, but different bacteria formed different colonies. With this method, the medical world finally had a truly objective way to distinguish among various bacterial types. In this way, physicians could begin to identify bacteria and associate a specific bacterial type with a particular disease. Koch's contributions to this budding field did not stop there. He went on to show that a single type of bacterium, isolated and reinoculated into animals, produced the same disease that afflicted animals from which it had come. He is credited with identifying and proving that cholera was caused by a comma-shaped bacterium he had discovered and that tuberculosis was caused by the tubercle bacillus, which he also isolated. This was solid proof of the role of these bacteria in these diseases and that only one bacterial type could produce a myriad of signs and symptoms involving multiple organs.

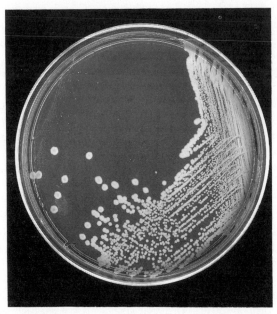

Figure 2.1. This is a modern-day version of the gelatin/agar plate originally developed by Robert Koch in 1881. It is used for the isolation and enumeration of bacteria. Each visible colony, a dot on the plate, represents hundreds of millions of progeny of a single bacterium that landed on the plate prior to overnight incubation.

BACTERIA AND THE DIVERSE MICROBIAL WORLD

Bacteria are independently multiplying microscopic single-cell organisms. We can safely state that, unlike angels, thousands can sit on the head of a pin. While we can see them under a 1000-fold magnification of the microscope (Figure 2.2), even at this enlargement they resemble specks, the size of small dust particles that we see dancing in front of headlights or around illuminated light

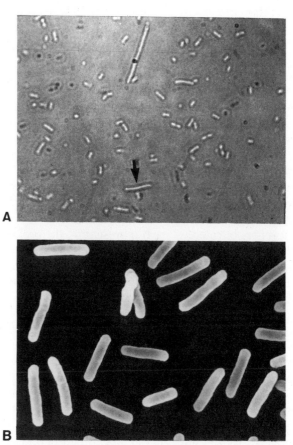

Figure 2.2. A) *Escherichia coli* bacteria visualized at approximately 1000-fold magnification under the phase microscope. Arrow points to one bacterium seen from its side. They appear as small moving spots in a fluid medium. B) *E. coli* under 3000-fold magnification by a scanning electron microscope (J. T. Park, Tufts University School of Medicine). The rod shape is typical of this intestinal bacterium.

bulbs. Under much higher magnification, such as with an electron microscope, they are seen much more clearly. One million bacteria are still invisible in a milliliter of liquid. Only when 10–100 million bacteria are present does the liquid become turbid.

Bacteria multiply by simple division, making a copy of their single chromosome and giving it to their progeny. Under the best laboratory conditions, growing in nutrient-rich media without competing predators, many types of bacteria can double their number within 20 minutes. In nature, they multiply less rapidly, often taking days to duplicate, since needed energy-producing materials are scarce and they are constantly in competition with neighboring microorganisms. For example, in the intestinal tract and on the skin, bacteria probably double no more than once every 12 to 24 hours. Although they can live as independent individual cells, they generally do not do so in nature. Instead, they exist in large numbers of colonies, each representing the progeny of a single cell, such as seen on Koch's gelatin agar plates. As colonies, they live in the intestinal tract and on the skin. There they are referred to as our "intestinal flora" and "skin flora" or microbiota. They also reside on soil particles in natural soils and in the sludge at the bottom of lakes, streams, and oceans. As groups of individual living entities, bacteria work together in a microscopic society, like ants in their ant hills, to obtain nutrients for growth and for survival of their population against the competition of other bacteria and predatory microorganisms. In this way, bacteria can also be likened to animal cells that work together as an interactive unit in the body to perform a particular function, such as the cells making up our heart, kidneys, and liver.

A single bacterium does no damage in nature and has little chance of survival. It must produce a large number of progeny in order to have any impact. Millions of bacteria are needed to produce enough toxins to cause disease or to digest enough tissue to lead to destruction of our internal organs, such as the intestine, lungs, or liver. Billions of bacteria are needed in order for them to become a stable component of an ecosystem, be it a soil or water niche, and even more of them to become the predominant form of bacteria in that ecological niche. About 10^{14} (one hundred thousand billion) bacteria live on the skin and in the gut of a human being. This amount is about ten times more than all the tissue cells that make up an average 150-pound person. Thus, although not seen, bacteria represent a major component of our body.

Scientists distinguish individual bacteria by their shapes—some are spherical, some are rodlike—and by the way they stain with a particular chemical preparation called the Gram stain. This method was discovered by Hans Christian Gram of Denmark in the late 1880s. He saw a color difference among bacteria that were contaminating a tissue preparation that he had stained with specific dyes in order to look for damages to the tissue. He noted that, in some samples, bacteria became colored a deep purple by the stain and retained this color during washing. These were designated "stain positive." Others lost the stain and were able to be counterstained with another, lighter dye and were colored pink; these he called "stain negative." In a survey of all forms of bacteria, this simple staining process proved readily useful for identifying different bacteria and placing them into one of two groups. Today this method has become a major way of distinguishing bacteria that are classified as either "Gram-positive" or "Gram-negative" (Table 2.1).

The Gram stain distinction derives from the differing composition of bacterial cell walls. Gram-negative bacteria, such as the common rod-shaped *Escherichia coli*, which are normal inhabitants of our guts, have a three-layer cell wall. The outer layer is made up of sugars attached to lipids; such a cell wall does not hold onto the Gram stain. The outer layer can be peeled away with appropriate dissolving agents, revealing a middle layer made mostly of protein. This middle layer maintains the cell's normal structure. Next to this layer is an inner layer, which, like the outer, is composed mostly of lipids and protein. The outer layer protects the cell against hazardous environmental materials, and the inner layer helps the bacterium to accumulate the materials it needs for energy and to excrete the materials that are toxic. Other common Gram-negative bacteria are shaped like tiny spheres or cocci.

Table 2.1. Bacteria and some common diseases.

Microorganism	Common Name	Disease
Gram Stain Positive		
Streptococcus pneumoniae	Pneumococcus	Lobar (pneumococcal) pneumonia Earache (otitis media)
Staphylococcus aureus	Golden staph	Septicemia Skin boils
Enterococcus faecalis	Enterococcus	Septicemia
Gram Stain Negative		
Neisseria meningitidis	Meningococcus	Meningitis
Neisseria gonorrhoeae	Gonococcus	Gonorrhea
Hemophilus influenzae	H. flu	Earache (otitis media) Pneumonia
Escherichia coli	Colibacillus	Urinary tract infection

These include the gonococcus and meningococcus, which can cause common infectious diseases.

The Gram-positive bacteria include the rod-shaped soil bacilli, which are not associated with human disease, and the round-shaped streptococci and staphylococci, which live on the skin and in the mouth. These bacteria have only a single cell wall made up of a proteinlike material combined with a lipid. This layer allows the cells to hold onto the color in the Gram stain during washing. It is this single layer, like the inner layer of Gram-negative bacteria, that performs uptake and excretion functions necessary for cell viability (Figure 2.3).

As with all of us, bacteria also need nutrients to survive. They live on simple environmental sources of the basic ingredients of matter—carbon, oxygen, hydrogen, and nitrogen. They obtain these by ingesting simple sugars located in the environment, by incorporating elements such as oxygen and nitrogen from the atmosphere into their diet, or by converting larger organic mate-

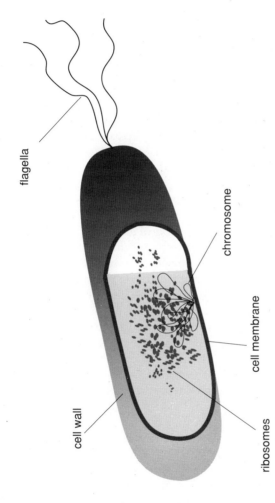

flagella

cell wall

ribosomes

cell membrane

chromosome

Figure 2.3. Diagram of an *E. coli* bacterium and its major components. Note the multilayered exterior consisting of an inner cell membrane and an outer cell wall, a single DNA chromosome, flagella that help it move, and ribosomes, sites of protein synthesis (Bonnie Marshall, Tufts University School of Medicine).

rials into needed substances. Some bacteria have special proteins, called enzymes, that can degrade organic matter into smaller nutritious elements. Others have the ability to break down complicated mixtures of fats or oils and live on the resultant enzymatically released nutrients. This is fortunate for us, since they are uniquely responsible for degrading organic wastes and for keeping our soils rich in nutrients for plant growth and agricultural products needed for human food production. They also can destroy toxic elements. The latter ability is presently being investigated as a future approach to the worldwide problem of environmental pollution. To help clean up toxic substances, bacteria that can degrade the harmful materials are being considered for purposeful release into polluted environments. An example is the use of "oil-eating" bacteria to help clean up the oil spill following the Exxon Valdez catastrophe a few years ago in Alaska.

Among the many different kinds of bacteria existing in our environment, there are those capable of living only in the presence of air (aerobic) and only in the absence of air (anaerobic). Some can live under either condition. For instance, *E. coli*, which live outside in the environment as well as inside our intestinal tract, can survive and grow under aerobic or anaerobic conditions. On the other hand, *Clostridium botulinum*, the microorganism that releases the deadly toxin causing botulism, can survive only anaerobically. Air is toxic to this and other purely anaerobic microorganisms. Anaerobic bacteria are particularly active in compost pits, where they turn refuse into reusable nutrients for other living matter.

Bacteria are also an essential part of our digestive tract, where they, along with stomach and pancreatic juices, help to digest unabsorbed food residues as they move through our large intestines before their final exits in the excreta. This digestion releases important nutrients and vitamins needed for our growth and well-being that can then be absorbed from our intestines into our bodies. Bacteria line our skin with a protective coat of defense against invasion by more harmful varieties of microorganisms. In these and other ways, we rely on many varieties of bacteria to help us survive in the natural environment.

BACTERIA AND DISEASE

Bacteria can also be described on the basis of their ability to cause disease: those harmful to humans, animals, or plants are called "pathogenic," and those relatively harmless are designated "nonpathogenic." However, this designation must also include an understanding of the host involved, since the same bacteria may be harmless to humans but harmful to other animals or plants, or vice versa. *Hemophilus influenzae* type b is a pathogen in humans, but not in animals. *Actinobacillus pleuropneumoniae* causes pneumonia in pigs but not in mankind. *Salmonella typhi*, the cause of typhoid fever, is pathogenic only in humans. Other salmonellae can cause disease, chiefly diarrheas, in mankind and animals. The basis of pathogenicity is the ability of bacteria to cause an infection—a form of destruction of an organ. Normally, an infection requires from tens of thousands to millions of bacteria to generate disease. Given these restraints, most bacteria entering our bodies by chance are quickly disarmed by our bodies' defenses and are unable to produce progeny. Among the most pathogenic bacteria, only 10 to 100 of them need to enter somewhere into our body to cause an infection. Disease occurs when bacteria multiply to high numbers before they can be removed or killed. Even one tubercle bacillus can cause tuberculosis if it enters and finds a protected site in the body of a susceptible person where it is able to multiply.

Each of us has natural defenses against bacterial invasion (Figure 2.4). One of our major defense organs is the skin. A similar role is played by the mucous membranes that line our mouth, intestines, and outlets of the bladder and genital tracts. Mucus secretions bathe these cells, preventing bacteria from adhering to them. Some secretions even have antibacterial activity, such as lysozyme found in tears. Cells lining our noses also contain threadlike hairs called cilia, which keep bacteria and other foreign objects from entering our upper respiratory passages and lungs.

If the skin is damaged, bacteria can enter through the cut and

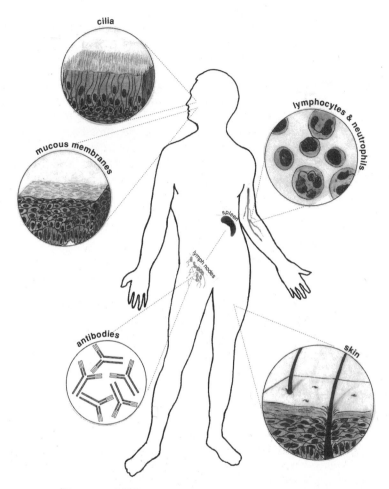

Figure 2.4. The human body has natural defenses against invasion by bacteria. These include the skin, mucous membranes lining the mouth and alimentary canal, cilia in the nasal passages, white blood cells, antibodies, and the reticulo-endothelial system consisting of connective tissue cells that remove foreign objects, such as bacteria. They line the blood sinusoids of liver, spleen, bone marrow, and lymph channels in lymph nodes (Bonnie Marshall, Tufts University School of Medicine).

then into the bloodstream, where they are disseminated to the rest of the body. Once past the skin, however, they face a second line of defense—circulating white blood cells ready to ingest and kill all invaders. The white cell response is helped by antibodies made against the invading organism. These antibodies help locate the foreign bacterium, attract white cell destroyers to it, or bring the organism to the spleen or lymph nodes, where it is destroyed. If the foreign invader can escape or overwhelm the white cells, it can grow to substantial enough numbers to cause real harm.

Some bacteria have intrinsic traits that can help them escape white cells. The composition of the bacterial outer cell wall is one of these. If it is rough or bulky in consistency, the bacterium is more easily engulfed by white blood cells. If it is smooth or slippery, however, the bacterium can evade the attack and ingestion more easily, giving it a better chance to reach areas in the body where it can settle and multiply to sufficient numbers to cause disease. Other cell wall changes allow bacteria to avoid recognition by the white cells, or allow them to survive ingestion. To thwart the host defense more, some bacteria can actually survive and multiply *within* the white cell. Such is the case for the *Legionella* bacterium that causes the acute respiratory disease now known as Legionnaire's Disease. (It got its name from the epidemic of respiratory disease and deaths at the American Legion Convention in Philadelphia in 1976.) The bacterium *Mycobacterium tuberculosis*, which causes tuberculosis, also lives in cells, making it particularly difficult to treat. The bacteria causing plague and typhoid fever also live and reproduce in human cells. These kinds of microorganisms must be eliminated quickly from the body before they take up residence in the very defense systems designed to destroy them.

Another important trait carried by some pathogenic bacteria is the ability to attach and grow on the surface of tissue cells that make up the animal or plant being invaded. This "colonization" ability allows them to withstand the movement of body fluids, such as urine and feces. While attached to these cells, the bacteria take in nutrients released from the animal cells. These nutrients are necessary for survival of the attached bacteria and for the production of their offspring.

The unfavorable interactions of bacteria with our defense systems are enhanced when bacteria can synthesize substances toxic to human tissues. Such substances may be enzymes that can digest the walls of human cells on which they are attached, or they may be toxins that can rapidly kill the cells. Toxin-producing bacteria cause the uncomfortable and sometimes severe diarrhea we encounter when traveling to certain parts of the world. They are an unsuspected part of the food we eat there. So-called traveller's diarrhea is, in large part, caused by toxin-producing bacteria in uncooked foods that reach our intestinal tracts and produce the toxins that irritate and kill intestinal cells. Our intestinal tract responds by contracting vigorously, an action we know as cramps. There is typically a release of large amounts of fluid, as an attempt to eliminate the toxin and the toxin-producing bacteria. Eventually these bacterial invaders are lost or replaced by more acceptable, nontoxin-producing strains in the environment. Or, more favorably, we recover our own intestinal bacterial microbiota after we return home.

It may not seem logical that the local inhabitants don't chronically, or even periodically, suffer from these diarrhea-causing bacteria. Some do; but most do not. To some extent, these local people have established an intestinal flora that is adapted to the local bacteria and so they are less affected than are visitors who arrive bearing their own, different flora. Local people also know what foods to avoid, something many visitors do not.

Scientifically, bacteria are only carrying out their own normal functions when they chance to find themselves inside an animal host. They have no purpose in invading, nor does invasion usually involve great numbers of bacteria. A few harmful bacteria may get into the body through a cut in the skin or a small opening in the mucous membranes. A few pathogens are ingested in foods, but most never get a hold on our bodies. Those intruding bacteria that escape detection and removal, however, thrive in excess nutrients. They form holes or abscesses in organs by releasing their destructive enzymes. We can most easily recognize this process when our body emits pus, which is a combination both of live and dead bacteria and of our own white cells that have arrived to destroy the bacteria.

The major energetic thrust of all microorganisms is to live and multiply. Yet should bacteria attack a vital organ—the heart, lung, or liver—they have ironically signed their own death warrants. In killing the person, the bacteria have, in fact, destroyed their life preserver and eventually die or are destroyed with the victim. This fatal and unwanted event differs dramatically from, say, a lion killing its prey for the food that will help it thrive. Microorganisms follow the biblical word to "live and multiply." Doing so, however, can lead to their own eventual demise.

OTHER MICROORGANISMS

Many types of microscopic single-cell microorganisms exist in nature (Figure 2.5). Some, such as those discussed already, are classified as bacteria because they are single-cell organisms and have no defined nuclei. Other examples of this type are the spirochetes and rickettsiae, which differ in size, shape, and genetic makeup from other bacteria. Taxonomists consider certain other single-cell microorganisms to be related more closely to animal and plant cells because they have a defined nucleus and other intracellular structures. These microorganisms include the yeasts, such as *Candida* or "monilia," and the fungi, which are of vastly different types. Only some of these are pathogenic to humans.

Viruses are much smaller than bacteria. Ten thousand of them can exist within a single cell. They are not independent microorganisms but are dependent on the host cell in order to produce copies of themselves. They consist of genetic material, DNA or RNA, enveloped in a protein coat. They are specialized in the sense that they attach to a specific structure on the particular host cell. They then inject their single, small piece of nucleic acid,

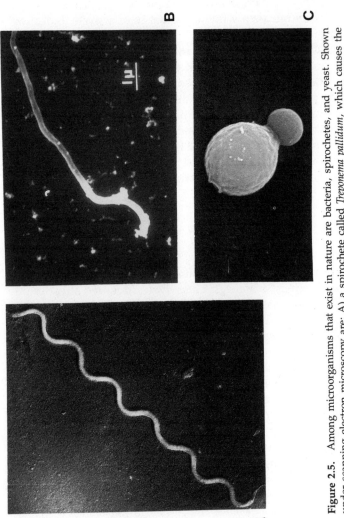

Figure 2.5. Among microorganisms that exist in nature are bacteria, spirochetes, and yeast. Shown under scanning electron microscopy are: A) a spirochete called *Treponema pallidum*, which causes the venereal disease syphilis (magnified 1300-fold) (James Miller, University of California, Los Angeles, California); B) *Borrelia bergendorfii*, a bacterium that causes Lyme disease (about 600-fold magnified) (Alan Steere, New England Medical Center, Boston); and C) *Candida albicans*, a common cause of yeast infection (magnified about 3500-fold) (David Soll, University of Iowa, Iowa City, Iowa).

which interrupts the function of the cell. The cell either dies or becomes a factory in the production of thousands of copies of the virus. Virologists have identified a multitude of different viruses and many more are yet to be found. One virus causes the devastating disease AIDS; another causes warts; still another causes hepatitis (Figure 2.6). Still others cause the common flu and winter cold. The origins and roles of these viruses in nature are unknown. Some biologists suggest that their existence results from random evolutionary events that produced agents capable of living on whole cells. In any case, they now contribute to the balance of nature. If a cell population increases, so do the viruses that kill these cells. Eventually, the cell population decreases, providing fewer hosts for the virus. Viruses without hosts are lost—and the balance in nature is restored.

A natural struggle continues between microorganisms (for instance, bacteria) and macroorganisms (for example, humans) and between microorganisms and other microorganisms. This conflict has taken place over the millennia in which bacteria have existed. Bacteria caused tuberculosis in ancient Egypt, as evidenced by scars and damaged tissues seen in mummies. Passages in the Bible refer to a venereal scourge, now known as gonorrhea, and evidence for this and another venereal disease, syphilis, has been found in ancient Egyptian tombs.

Our inherent ability to survive bacterial invasion rests on our natural defenses, namely the production of antibodies and the activity of white cells. In the last half century, naturally occurring substances that aid in killing bacteria without harming the body have been added to these natural functions. These agents are the antibiotics.

DISCOVERY OF ANTIBIOTICS: ORIGINS AND SUCCESSES

With the acceptance of the germ theory of disease in the late 1800s came a change in the goals of treatment. An era began in

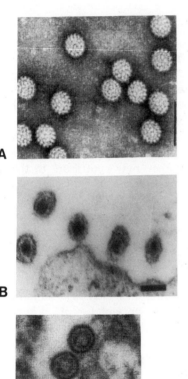

Figure 2.6. Shown here by electron microscopy (about 37,500-fold magnification) are three viruses implicated in human diseases: A) the wart virus, which causes the common human wart; B) HIV-1, the virus that causes AIDS; and C) HHV-6, a herpes-like virus associated with the childhood disease "erythemum subitum" (Jay Levy, University of California, San Francisco).

which physicians and scientists searched for drugs that would kill the disease-causing agent, the bacterium or the parasite. The outcome of this search was the almost serendipitous discovery of antibiotics.

That living beings produce substances that inactivate or kill others was first put forth under the heading of "antibiosis" by the

Frenchman, Paul Vuillemin, head of Natural History at the medical faculty of the University of Nancy. His description, presented in 1889, dealt with negative effects or interactions that affected survival among animals and among plants, not among bacteria. He spoke of these as "influences antibiotiques," that is "antibiotic influences." An antibiotic, as we now know it, is a natural substance made by one microorganism that inhibits growth of another microorganism. The actual term "antibiotic" is attributed to Selman Waksman, the American soil microbiologist and discoverer of the antibiotic streptomycin. He suggested the term in 1941 to the editor of *Biologic Abstracts* as a word for indexing a growing number of these kinds of antibacterial agents.

It would appear that antibiotics were inadvertently used even before their discovery. Ancient writings report the application of cloths impregnated with natural substances and other forms of organic matter onto wounds in order to help them heal. We suspect that these old remedies worked because they contained microorganisms producing antibiotics or the drugs themselves. Anthropologists have unearthed traces of the antibiotic tetracycline in thousand-year-old Nubian mummies. Microorganisms producing this antibiotic were found in soil samples that came from the same area where the mummies were discovered. Traces of tetracycline were recovered in grain as well. The Nubian nation survived a long time, from ancient times to the 14th century. Some scientists suggest that this long survival may in part be linked to the presence and use, either on purpose or by chance, of small amounts of crude antibiotics, such as the tetracyclines.

At the end of the 19th century, research scientists astutely put their energies into exploring methods that would use harmless bacteria to treat disease caused by harmful bacteria. Whole, harmless bacteria were fed to patients to compete with the harmful disease-causing ones in hopes that the harmless ones would win out. In Paris in 1877, Louis Pasteur, with his colleague Jules François Joubert, described how anthrax, a disease caused by a bacillus, was suppressed in animals that were injected with harmless soil bacteria. Ten years later the German scientist Rudolf

Emmerich noted that guinea pigs infected previously with a streptococcus were protected from developing cholera when injected with the cholera bacillus. He was the first to capitalize on this finding and use it to prevent cholera in animals.

About a year later in France, Charles Bouchard showed that injection of small amounts of *Pseudomonas aeruginosa* protected rabbits from contracting anthrax. In related events, other investigators noted that the typhoid fever bacillus survived longer when placed into sterile water than when introduced into water containing other organisms. All these findings implied a negative effect of the other bacteria on growth of these pathogenic bacteria. The basis for these findings was fully realized in retrospect only when antibiotics as products of bacteria were discovered.

Historic developments that aided in identifying and enumerating bacteria contributed greatly to the discovery of antibiotics. Perhaps principal among these was Robert Koch's gelatin-containing agar plate. Since investigators could grow and count bacteria in the laboratory following a single day, or night, of incubation, potential growth-inhibiting substances could be tested in the agar along with bacteria. If the bacteria grew, the substance was not active. If bacteria did not grow, the substance was a potential agent for treating disease caused by that bacterium.

The First Antibiotics

The first natural antibacterial product, that is, one that was not made by chemists and thus meriting the designation antibiotic, was pyocyanase, which rapidly gained international recognition. Its discovery in 1888 was partly serendipitous and partly the result of the search for these kinds of agents. E. de Freudenreich in Germany found that the blue pigment released in the broth culture of the blue-pus bacterium, *Bacillus pyocyaneus* (now known as *P. aeruginosa*), stopped the growth of other bacteria in the test tube. This activity suggested that the bacteria were producing a potentially useful agent to treat human disease caused by bacteria susceptible to this material.

Rudolf Emmerich, who had previously focused on microbe–microbe interactions, joined with Oscar Loew, also from Germany, to investigate this phenomenon further. They confirmed the previous findings and named the substance "pyocyanase" after the producing bacterium, adding "ase" because they considered the activity to be that of an enzyme protein. (It was shown later to be made of a lipid.) They performed the first extensive clinical trials of pyocyanase in 1889. Their reports lauded the beneficial effects of the drug, not only in inhibiting bacterial growth, but also in actually killing pathogenic bacteria, including those causing typhoid fever, anthrax, diphtheria, plague, and skin abscesses. The discovery was followed with great interest and excitement since it heralded a major breakthrough. When it came to applying these laboratory results to the patient, however, pyocyanase lost its luster. It was toxic and unstable. It was not the lifesaving potion they had sought. Still, its use persisted for almost thirty years, mainly as a topical ointment on the skin. By 1913, reports about any therapeutic efficacy of pyocyanase had almost disappeared.

Paul Ehrlich, a chemist working in Berlin, took a different approach. He was fascinated by dyes that stained tissues and microorganisms. He reasoned that such selectivity could help find a "magic bullet," that is, a substance that rids the body selectively of the infecting microorganism, whether it be a bacterium or parasite, without harming the body tissues. His first successful candidate product, reported in 1910, was the drug Salvarsan, a chemical dye linked to arsenic. Its discovery came out of his search for agents to treat the trypanosome parasite that causes African sleeping sickness. Salvarsan received its greatest recognition when it was shown to help patients afflicted with syphilis. The drug worked, but not uniformly, and the toxicity of the arsenic derivative subjected patients to severe and sometimes painful and debilitating side effects. Still, it was a breakthrough—the first direct treatment of this common disease. Its discovery opened the door to a new era of interest in chemotherapy. The early decades of the 20th century passed, however, without much advancement in the search for antibacterial substances. It is believed that the failure of pyocyanase and other candidates to live up to Ehrlich's "magic bullet" dream probably had a discouraging effect on the search for other compounds of this type. Reports surfaced of better antiseptics—agents that would sterilize surgical instruments and even certain skin wounds—but these could not be taken into the body. Many of these could not even be used on humans because they were toxic to the skin. Instead, they were relegated to disinfecting utensils, such as those used in surgery. None of these materials proved to be that magic substance that would be effective and nontoxic when taken internally. General enthusiasm for the ideal substance waned.

Discovery of Penicillin

Still, some laboratories persisted in the search. Alexander Fleming, working at St. Mary's Hospital in London, discovered and reported in the 1920s a naturally occurring antibacterial substance in human tears that caused certain bacterial cells to break open and die. He called this material "lysozyme," since it caused susceptible bacteria to fall apart or to lyse. Unfortunately, it too proved to have no practical place as a therapeutic agent. For one, its effectiveness was mostly limited to nonpathogenic bacteria and, additionally, it was not easily made in large enough amounts to allow for sufficient testing in people or animals. Its importance lay more in its being one of the first natural substances identified within humans with the real or potential role of protecting us against bacterial invasion.

In 1928, Fleming happened on his second antibacterial discovery—this time a major one. Coming back from a weekend vacation, he went through his usual routine of looking at some of the old plates that had been left in his work area. In doing so, he noticed a discarded plate that had not yet been submerged in a detergent solution. There he saw that colonies of the common skin organism *Staphylococcus* had lysed—fallen apart—seemingly by the product of a mold growing in the adjacent area. He observed that the lysis occurred only in this one area and showed that this

effect was caused by the mold that was growing next to the
bacterial colonies on the plate (Figure 2.7). Had this gelatin plate
been submerged into the detergent solution along with all the
others, which was the case for the majority of discarded plates,
this history-making discovery would not have been made, at least
not then.

As Fleming freely admitted, the interference with bacterial
growth by a fungus had been seen by many others before him,
but no one paid much attention to the phenomenon. In the late
1890s, a professor at Johns Hopkins University in Baltimore reportedly showed his students an agar plate on which a mold appeared
to be inhibiting the growth of bacteria isolated from urine. But the
significance of this observation was not appreciated—at least there

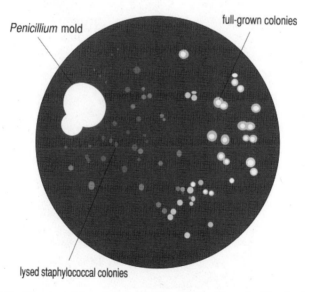

Figure 2.7. Diagram of the original plate observed by Alexander Fleming in 1928
showing lysis of staphylococcal colonies growing near a mold that happened to be
on the same plate (Bonnie Marshall, Tufts University School of Medicine).

was no apparent follow-up of the finding. But in retrospect, this event preceded Fleming's findings by thirty years, which were also those of serendipity and observation.

Fleming was fascinated by the phenomenon and guessed that he was witnessing an important medical breakthrough, the actual falling apart, or lysis, of already-formed colonies (Figure 2.8). Perhaps this also reminded him of his work on lysozyme that also caused lysis, although lysozyme's effect was on individual bacteria rather than on whole colonies. Being familiar with one kind of lytic agent, he happened upon another. This one came not from human fluids but was presumably made by the mold on the plate.

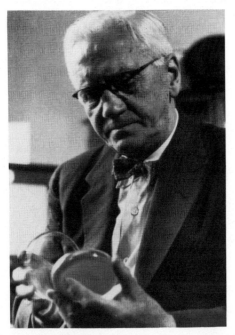

Figure 2.8. Alexander Fleming (1881–1955), who discovered penicillin in 1928 (G. MacFarlane, *Alexander Fleming: The Man and the Myth*, Harvard University Press, Cambridge. Reprinted by permission).

Fleming soon demonstrated that, in fact, the mold made a substance small enough to diffuse through the agar and lyse the
bacteria. He called it "penicillin" after the *Penicillium* mold that had
produced it. By extracting the substance from cultures of the
mold, he was able to show its antibacterial activity directly. Penicillin was so uniquely active that small amounts of culture fluids
could produce this killing effect. And, more importantly, it tri-
umphed over a very common and deadly bacterium, *Staphylococcus aureus*, which caused skin infections, often leading to
blood-borne dangerous septic disease. The events surrounding
Fleming's discovery have challenged historians and microbiologists trying to reproduce the exact conditions that led to his seeing
this lytic event on the agar plates. Still, the proof of the happening
lies in the dried original plate that Fleming kept and remains in the
archives at St. Mary's Hospital in London.

Prontosil: Revival of Interest in Antibiotics

Fleming is credited with discovering our first true antibiotic,
penicillin. While the discovery was made in 1928, use of penicillin
as a therapeutic agent to treat infections in humans did not occur
until the 1940s. Fleming attributed this delay to a lack of biochemical and microbiological expertise at the time. There also existed at
that time a mentality that discouraged the possibility of finding
substances that could be used internally to treat major infectious
diseases. As we mentioned before, this lack of initiative was
probably the legacy of the failure of pyocyanase and the toxicity of
Salvarsan. But an event in the 1930s turned this attitude around.

Gerhard Domagk, director of research at I. G. Farbenindus-
trie in Germany, was examining different chemical dyes for their
effect on bacterial infections. In the course of these studies, he
discovered an antibacterial agent that worked when given to
animals. This was not an antibiotic in the true sense of the word,
since it was man-made and not a natural product. Like penicillin,
its discovery occurred somewhat by accident. Domagk found that

Prontosil, a newly patented dye, cured diseases caused by the streptococcus bacteria when injected into diseased mice. He had been motivated to try dyes as antimicrobials because he knew that they stained bacteria as well as tissues, and he reasoned that perhaps, when taken up by the bacteria, they would interfere with growth. It is interesting to note that Domagk and colleagues tested all the chemicals, including Prontosil, in animals as well as test tubes. Had he relied only on the test tube assay, his discovery would never have been made.

Prontosil was active only when put into mice and not when tested against growing bacteria in a test tube—an unusual finding not observed for any other previously described agent. The answer to this mystery came later. Others discovered that it was not the dye part of the molecule but the chemical attached to it, the sulfonamide portion, that when released during metabolism of the compound in the body, killed the bacteria.

It was the effectiveness of Prontosil, and later other sulfonamide derivatives, which scientists regard as the critical event leading to the resurgence of interest in antibiotics. At long last, physicians had an agent that, when taken internally, worked and was nontoxic and stable. The results of pyocyanase and other ineffective agents were relegated to ancient history. This discovery created a new receptive atmosphere for the development and production of penicillin, which had already been discovered seven years before Domagk's eventful experiments with Prontosil. There was renewed interest in discovering other "magic bullets." Some were to be newly discovered; other potential agents were being reexamined in a new, more optimistic light.

The Search for Antibiotics

With the successes of sulfonamides known widely, the quest for other forms of antibacterial agents revived. Common soil dug up from anywhere in the ground became the focus of these new searches. As far back as the 1890s, Robert Koch, the inventor of the gelatin plate, was fascinated by the fact that pathogenic bacteria died when put into soil. He wondered why. A half century later, in the 1940s, Selman Waksman and other soil microbiologists went back to examine the same phenomenon. They searched in hopes of finding the inhibitors of bacterial growth in the soil, notably among the soil microorganisms themselves.

Waksman said at a meeting of the National Academy of Sciences in Washington in 1940:

> Bacteria pathogenic to man and animals find their way to the soil, either in the excreta of the hosts or in their remains. If one considers the period for which animals and plants have existed on this planet and the great numbers of disease-producing microbes that must have thus gained entrance into the soil, one can only wonder that the soil harbors so few bacteria capable of causing infectious diseases in man and animals. . . . It was suggested that the cause of the disappearance of these disease-producing organisms in the soil is to be looked for among the soil-inhabiting microbes, antagonistic to the pathogens and bringing about their rapid destruction in the soil.[1]

On the basis of these considerations, Waksman and others went to the soil, "panning" for these antagonistic substances. Their work did not go unrewarded. Their activities not only advanced the science of soil microbiology, but also led to the golden age of antibiotic discovery.

Waksman's suppositions and interpretations in the 1940s grew out of a long period of experiments in soil microbiology that he had begun several decades before. This initial work had focused on the discovery of bacteria as sources of enzymes for chemical processes. His new efforts once again generated great interest in the soil for different kinds of substances, namely those that could cure infections.

Therefore, it is perhaps not surprising that one of Waksman's former students, René J. Dubos, a graduate of the French National Institute of Agronomy in Paris who worked with Waksman on his prior research, turned to the soil in his search for antibiotics. In 1939, while at the Rockefeller Institute, Dubos isolated, for the first time, an antibiotic-producing soil microorganism. His discovery also led to the first clinically useful antibiotic, beating the discovery of penicillin by about five years. By mixing the infectious bacteria *Staphylococcus* with cultures of different soil bacteria, Dubos noticed one culture that would not allow growth of the staphylococci. In this successful culture, he identified a *Bacillus brevis* bacterium that excreted a substance into the culture fluid that killed the staphylococci. Because this substance only seemed to kill the Gram-positive organisms—that group of bacteria identified by their ability to take up the stain developed by Gram—he named it "gramicidin." Dubos presented his discovery to the world at the International Congress of Microbiology in New York in 1940. Following on the heels of the synthetic sulfonamides, gramicidin was the first natural product extracted from a soil organism and shown to have these antibacterial properties. But the drug had certain major drawbacks, in particular, a severe toxicity when given intravenously. Still, gramicidin found a place in human therapy as an external application for minor skin infections, a purpose for which it is still used today.

Development of Penicillin

On the other side of the Atlantic, a team led by the English pathologist Howard Florey was responsible for the renewed interest in finding more antibiotics. Encouraged by the successes of sulfonamides, Florey decided to put together a team to evaluate antibacterials. He was soon joined by Ernst Chain, a German-born biochemist with whom he would collaborate for years. They began their experiments in the late 1930s and continued into the fifth decade. After a search of the literature for potential substances, they decided to begin with lysozyme. But after several years they realized that this was not the agent to be pursued. They moved to another of Fleming's agents, penicillin. They were working in Oxford, not far from London, where Fleming was still located at St. Mary's Hospital. While Fleming had continued to work on penicillin, he was not able to purify enough of it to test in animals or humans.

For penicillin, then, it was Florey and Chain who became the clear flag bearers. They and their colleagues learned how to extract the substance, how to keep it stable, and how to produce it in amounts sufficient to test in animals. Their results were spectacular. Mice destined to die from infection were miraculously cured by this drug. When sufficient quantities were made to test in people, the limited amounts available were used only on very sick patients whose infectious disease had reached near fatal proportions. Use of even very small amounts of penicillin, in a crude state, was able to turn the tide of the infection and cure individuals considered to be on their death beds. In some instances, the drug was so scarce that any of it that came out in the patients' urine was reextracted and used for subsequent doses!

The small amounts of penicillin were only enough to treat a limited number of patients; however, joint efforts by Florey and his colleagues, along with American physicians and scientists, as well as the trials following the Cocoanut Grove fire, convinced United States pharmaceutical firms and the United States government to begin producing it in large quantities. Using an unusual form of intraindustry cooperation, several companies accelerated the scale of production. Initially, penicillin was reserved exclusively to treat soldiers and a few lucky civilians. It more or less "belonged" to the military. Eventually, by 1944, penicillin became available to the public. With its widespread use came more publicity, this time, staggering. Fleming was called "one of the great scientists of the 20th century." His picture was featured on the May 15, 1944, cover of *Time* magazine. Without the revelatory power of television, with only newsreels, radio, and newspapers, the thrilling story of the miracle of penicillin was told and retold to audiences around the world.

Soon, the discovery of penicillin took on mythic proportions. It was as if Prometheus had stolen fire from the gods. The applications of this wonder drug seemed all but limitless. In fact, people began to assume that it could cure and help any disease. Even within the medical literature of the time, we can find passages stating that penicillin had worked on cancers and on viral infections—diseases and conditions for which we now know penicillin has no effect. These distorted expectations became a part of the mystique surrounding penicillin and other antibiotics, which has been carried over even into present times. To many, an antibiotic is a "cure-all" to be taken for any illness, though, in fact, it can treat only certain illnesses. In the 1940s there was no way to control what was being said or thought about penicillin. Penicillin became whatever people wanted it to be. Faced with the ravages of war, people needed something to pin their hopes on. To some degree, penicillin played that role and public consensus mandated that the drug be available to everyone.

Streptomycin: A Cure for Tuberculosis

The first major breakthrough in the search for an internally useful antibiotic from soil was made in 1943 by Selman Waksman and his group working at the New Jersey State Agriculture Experimental Station at Rutgers University. Aware of the discovery of gramicidin by Dubos, Waksman had already turned his attention away from enzymes produced by soil bacteria and began to look for those making antibiotics. From over 10,000 cultures of potential producers, Waksman and his colleagues, in collaboration with Merck and Company in nearby Rahway, New Jersey, selected ten microorganisms that seemed to hold the most promise. Among these was *Streptomyces griseus*. This producer proved to be different from any of the other microorganisms previously found to make antibiotics. It was neither a mold nor a member of the *Bacillus* group of bacteria, such as the one that made gramicidin. It was a member of another family of soil bacteria, the actinomycetes. The antibiotic that *S. griseus* produced was subsequently called "streptomycin."

Streptomycin proved effective not only in the test tube, but also in people. It was active against bacteria that caused common infections, such as urinary tract infections, and against those causing meningitis; it also was effective in combatting more unusual ones, like the systemic disease tularemia, which is spread by infected animals and ticks. Yet its most acclaimed use was discovered when it was found to kill the then untouchable bacterium *Mycobacterium tuberculosis*, the cause of tuberculosis. This was the first antibiotic or drug of any kind that offered hope to victims suffering from this chronic, debilitating, and often fatal disease.

Streptomycin, however, triggered certain side effects that were not observed with penicillin. Streptomycin, in the accumulated dosage needed to cure the disease, could cause damage to the kidneys and lead to temporary and even persistent deafness. Attempts to modify it chemically in order to reduce its toxicity were not successful. A second problem proved to be even more critical, namely that during therapy, bacteria became resistant to the killing effect of streptomycin at a frequency that compromised treatment. This phenomenon did not occur very easily with the antibiotics penicillin or gramicidin. Although penicillin-resistant bacteria existed, their numbers were small and they did not pose a great clinical dilemma. Mutants did not appear during drug therapy as they did with streptomycin.

The rapid emergence of mutants resistant to streptomycin encouraged the Merck laboratories and other groups to look for other antibiotics that were both safer than streptomycin and to which spontaneous resistance was less likely to occur. The fruit of these efforts was the antibiotic neomycin, to which bacteria did not develop resistance so easily. The drug was also very toxic, however. It is used today primarily in topical antibacterial ointments. Neomycin is related structurally to streptomycin and became the second in this "aminoglycoside" group of antibiotics to which were later added the antibiotics kanamycin (1957), gentamicin (1963), tobramycin (1971), and amikacin, a semisynthetic derivative of kanamycin. These latter antibiotics have proven very useful as systemic treatment agents.

THE BIRTH OF BROAD SPECTRUM AGENTS

Chloramphenicol

Other drugs still in use today also made their appearance at the end of the 1940s. A Yale University microbiologist, Paul Burkholder, was conducting his own search for antibiotic-producing microorganisms in soils that he had obtained from many different countries. When he found microorganisms that produced substances that inhibited the growth of other bacteria, he would send them to the Parke Davis Company in Detroit for confirmation and additional testing. In the summer of 1947, he discovered one microorganism, from a soil sample collected in a field in Caracas, Venezuela, that produced an inhibitory substance that appeared to kill a wide variety of bacterial types. The diversity of bacteria affected made the discovery exciting and novel. Burkholder extended his studies with the microorganism to more and more different kinds of bacteria and found that the drug was the first discovered that inhibited both Gram-positive and Gram-negative bacteria, that is, bacteria with very different cell wall structures as distinguished by the Gram stain. The compound was named Chloromycetin, based on the fact that it contained a chlorine atom (chloro) and was produced by a member of the actinomycete (mycin) family, and later named *Streptomyces venezuela* after its country of origin.

Chloromycetin, also known as the chemical substance chloramphenicol, rose to prominence when investigators discovered that its spectrum of activity included members of a different type of bacterial group, the rickettsiae. These infectious agents, carried by ticks and other mites, cause epidemic typhus and Rocky Mountain Spotted Fever, both potentially fatal diseases. The first human trial of chloramphenicol came in La Paz, Bolivia, where public health officials were trying to cope with an epidemic of typhus. Parke Davis sent down as much of the chloramphenicol as they could. Fourteen of the fifty patients for whom there was no chloramphenicol died, but all twenty-two who were treated, recovered.

Having identified both a new antibiotic and the cure of a previously untreatable disease, investigators went on to test the effect of the drug against other bacteria. They found that chloramphenicol was also very effective in the treatment of the bacterium that causes typhoid fever. These bacteria were not susceptible to any antibiotic known at the time.

The success of chloramphenicol, however, was marred by the discovery that the drug had potentially life-threatening toxic side effects. A small percentage of treated patients (now known to be about one in 40,000) suffered from bone marrow suppression causing the loss of circulating red cells and white cells. A smaller number went on to irreversible total bone marrow collapse leading to anemias and even leukemias. As a consequence, the United States and other countries decided it was too risky to keep chloramphenicol as a first-line therapy for any disease. In special instances it is still used today, notably for serious illnesses that have not responded to other antibiotics. In the developing world, however, despite its toxicity, chloramphenicol is used extensively to treat severe diarrheas and pneumonias. This practice continues because the drug is so inexpensive and, therefore, more easily affordable in areas where the cost of substitute drugs precludes their widespread use. Another rationale for its use would be the suspicion that the patient with diarrhea could have typhoid fever, for which chloramphenicol remains a drug of choice.

The Tetracyclines

Chloramphenicol was the first of the class of "broad spectrum" antibiotics. Its reserved use, because of toxicity, was probably facilitated by the finding of other antibiotics with wide antimicrobial activity.

At the same time that Burkholder was studying chloramphenicol, Benjamin Duggar, at the Lederle Laboratories in Pearl River, New York, became fascinated by a microorganism that excreted a golden-colored substance that had novel antibiotic properties. The microorganism, now called *Streptomyces aureofaciens*, produced the antibiotic then called aureomycin and now known as chlortetracycline, the first member of the tetracycline family of antibiotics. The drug, introduced in 1948, showed low toxicity and a broad spectrum of activity against bacteria. Both features propelled it to worldwide use within one to two years of its introduction into the clinical arena. It also proved effective against rickettsiae and the typhoid bacillus as well as a long list of other disease-causing bacteria, making it a clear alternative to the more toxic chloramphenicol. By 1955, only seven years after chlortetracycline was introduced, over 8,000 papers were already published describing its use in both acute and chronic infections. Its eventual low price and broad spectrum of activity have made it a commonly used antibiotic in the developing world. Today tetracyclines rank second only to penicillins in world production and world use.

Following the discovery of these first-generation antibiotics, more antibiotics were discovered, tested, and introduced with unprecedented rapidity. These events occurred in countries all over the world during the decades of the 1950s, 1960s, and early 1970s (Table 2.2).

THE CEPHALOSPORINS: OTHER PENICILLINLIKE ANTIBIOTICS WITH BROAD SPECTRUM ACTIVITY

Two unique pencillinlike drugs, cephalothin and cephaloridine, were introduced in 1964. The time from discovery to entry into the clinical arena was much longer than with previous antibiotics. The initial discovery leading to the development of these drugs came in 1945 by the Italian microbiologist Giuseppe Brotsu. He noticed antibacterial activity in extracts from a mold he found in a sewer outlet off the coast of Sardinia. It took years to purify the active agent. He sent his materials to Florey and researchers at Oxford who found a number of different antibiotics in the culture fluid. Once the chemical structure of the most active component

Table 2.2. Chronology of antimicrobial discovery and clinical use (1929–1972).

	Event	Country
1929	penicillin discovered	England
1932	sulfonamides (Prontosil) discovered	Germany
1939	gramicidin discovered	United States
1942	penicillin introduced	England and United States
1943	streptomycin discovered	United States
1943	bacitracin discovered	United States
1945	cephalosporins discovered	Italy
1947	chloramphenicol discovered	United States
1947	chlortetracycline discovered	United States
1949	neomycin discovered	United States
1950	oxytetracycline discovered	United States
1952	erythromycin discovered	United States
1956	vancomycin discovered	United States
1957	kanamycin discovered	Japan
1960	methicillin introduced	England and United States
1961	ampicillin introduced	England
1961	spectinomycin reported	United States
1963	gentamicin discovered	United States
1964	cephalosporins introduced	England
1966	doxycycline introduced	United States
1967	clindamycin reported	United States
1971	tobramycin discovered	United States
1972	cephamycins (cefoxitin) discovered	United States
1972	minocycline introduced	United States

was known, derivatives that were more stable and retained high and broad spectrum antibacterial activity were made. The two cephalosporins mentioned above were the fruits of these efforts. Three years later, in 1967, two orally effective cephalosporins were ready for clinical use. One of these, cephalexin, remains in high usage today. Continued modification of cephalosporins, as with penicillins, has led to more and more derivatives with properties varying in rate and extent of oral absorption, length of time of activity in the body, spectrum of activity and insensitivity to cephalosporin-degrading enzymes, the so-called cephalosporin-ases.

THE SYNTHETIC ANTIMICROBIALS

Added to the growing field of naturally occurring antibacterial substances were substances that were chemically synthesized. The first group of these was the sulfonamide family, whose successful use preceded all of the "natural" antibiotics. As effective as antibiotics are, these products were not naturally produced by other bacteria and consequently have been called synthetic antimicrobials, or just antimicrobials. Sulfonamide derivatives followed the discovery that the active antibacterial agent in Prontosil was in actuality a sulfonamide. These were synthesized in the 1930s and into the 1940s in many different forms, enlarging their spectrum of activity, their pharmacologic features (that is, the length of time they would reside in the body), and the method of inoculation, whether by injection or by mouth. The development of this group of highly effective drugs forms the foundation of this era of antimicrobial discovery and development. Today, sulfonamides represent a relatively large proportion (about 10%) of all antimicrobial agents being produced and sold throughout the world.

Trimethoprim was the second of the synthetic antimicrobials to take its place in the popular marketplace. Its introduction in the 1970s came in combination with a sulfonamide, sulfamethoxazole, in a single medication form called cotrimoxazole, for the treatment of Gram-negative and Gram-positive infections. It proved extremely effective against infectious microorganisms of the urinary tract and in systemic infections, such as those caused by *Salmonella*, *E. coli*, or *Hemophilus*. Its ability to penetrate deeply into tissues made it an alternative for the therapy of such diseases as typhoid fever, where the bacteria often "hide" in the gallbladder or within lymph nodes. The combination of trimethoprim and a sulfonamide was touted and advanced because it involved the use of two agents, both synthetic, and both of which acted on naturally occurring enzymes at different steps in a metabolic pathway essential to the growth of bacteria. It was assumed that resistance to two synthetic agents would not appear. That assumption may have held, had sulfonamide resistance not been already so prominent when this drug was introduced. In fact, it was shown that the high success rate of the combination drug was essentially linked to the trimethoprim itself. In a departure from the usual mode of introduction, trimethoprim, as a therapeutic alone, was later introduced, after it had already been used in combination with sulfonamides.

Recently, another group of synthetic agents has taken center stage. These drugs are related to an older synthetic agent, nalidixic acid. They have proven effective against a wide variety of Gram-positive and Gram-negative bacteria. The core of these agents is a chemical structure called a "quinolone," and thus they are called fluoroquinolones. In contrast to the rapid emergence of bacteria resistant to nalidixic acid, in a frequency resembling that of streptomycin, these new agents show an exceedingly lower tendency to select resistant mutants.

The fluoroquinolones can be taken by mouth and still achieve a high concentration in the blood stream. This feature permits excellent antibacterial coverage by the medication when taken at home, an advantage in this day of rising hospital costs. The quinolones are, in fact, being used as agents for treatment of infectious diseases that require prolonged therapy, of anywhere from several weeks to several months.

Given these advantages, that is, low toxicity and infrequent selection of resistant mutants, quinolones have become a popular new group of antimicrobial agents. More and more derivatives have appeared, and additional ones are still coming onto the market. Each derivative differs from the others in its time of circulation in the body and the group of microorganisms on which it is active. For instance, some derivatives have shown surprising efficacy against bacteria that have been traditionally difficult to treat, such as the bacteria causing leprosy.

Synthesis of Methicillin in Response
to Mounting Penicillin Resistance

Early in the antibiotic era, with the advent of oral and other noninjectible forms of penicillin, this valued agent began to be used in a large variety of over-the-counter preparations, including "salves, throat lozenges, nasal ointments, and even cosmetic creams"—all "marketed in response to the public clamor for the 'miracle drug'."[2]

By 1955, most countries restricted the use of penicillin to that by prescription only. But widespread usage had already occurred. This uncontrolled early usage led to a legacy of growing resistance in that decade and beyond, a widespread resistance to penicillin, especially among the staphylococci. Historically, a concerted effort was made by pharmaceutical houses to deal with this resistance, to try to circumvent the enzymatic degradation of this valued therapeutic agent.

An answer to the resistance problem came with the discovery and introduction of methicillin in the early 1960s. This semisynthetic penicillin was insensitive to the bacterial enzymes that degraded penicillin. Other derivatives able to be taken orally soon followed. While this advance initially stemmed the avalanche of penicillin resistance, it revealed yet another unwelcomed surprise—bacterial resistance to this semisynthetic drug itself, a problem now faced worldwide.

FUTURE ANTIBIOTICS

It is only in the present century, and more recently since the 1940s, that we have seen the rapid development and production of antibiotics. In 1949, the United States produced penicillin and streptomycin at a rate of 6.5 tons per month. In 1954, between 400,000 and 500,000 pounds of broad-spectrum antibiotics were being made. Today, the United States produces almost 40 million pounds annually. This figure alone tells us something about the growth of this industry.

The quest for new antibiotics continues, but at a slower pace. New drug discoveries too often come up with an antibiotic that is not really original but is a derivative member of a family already described. Chemical synthesis to modify antibiotics already in hand offers some approach to developing derivatives that are truly different. It is clear, however, that more initiatives to identify truly new antibiotics, and especially to safeguard the antibiotics we now have, are the goals for the next decade.

Chapter 3

RELIANCE ON MEDICINES AND SELF-MEDICATION

The Seeds of Antibiotic Misuse

Antibiotics are a medical treasure, perhaps the most important therapeutic discovery in the history of medicine. But they are being misused. In some cases, they are taken when they are not needed at all; in others, they are prescribed and used inappropriately. For example, they are given in too small or too large amounts or for too long or too short periods of time. The old adage applies here. "Too much of a good thing can be bad." In the case of antibiotics, we must add, "so can too little." Not only quantity, but length of usage, either too long or too short, can affect the therapeutic and environmental consequences of these agents.

Misuse has led to the decreased effectiveness of antibiotics because of the emergence of bacteria that are resistant to them. Antibiotics, like other pharmaceuticals, "suffer" from the present day reliance on medication to cure every ailment, the "pill for every ill" belief. In the quest for a rapid relief of symptoms, medicines that are freely available to people are being misused. So it is with antibiotics. They have been overused and used inappropriately, creating in their wake an environment where antibiotic-resistant bacteria survive.

Overreliance on medicine to treat an array of illnesses is not unique to antibiotics. It reflects humanity's understandable desire for relief from illness, the rush to use medicines in order to return to a normal daily life. This attitude, however, was not always so prominent. In early times, when medicinal substances were not plentiful, the power of the word and communication with the spirits played an important role. The inclusion of a nonmedicinal approach to therapy was retained for a long time during and after the discovery of effective medications. Eventually, however, the chant and the communication were replaced almost completely by medicines.

HISTORICAL OVERVIEW

A brief account of the history leading to modern-day medicine is worth noting, since it sets the background in which antibiotics were discovered and may help to explain society's current expectations and attitudes toward these drugs.

Early ancestors believed that each and every distinct "thing"—whether a tree, a stone, or a drinking vessel—was imbued with a spirit. When someone suddenly fell ill, it was assumed that an object was taking vengeance for a slight or grievance that had been committed against it—an unacceptable offering, a felled tree, an overturned stone. Suffering from headache, fever, stomach cramps, or aching muscles, the patient would seek out a healer to calm the spirits and dispel the symptoms. This healer, whether self-proclaimed or appointed, would proceed, as he and his forebears had done many times before, to address the "souls in conflict" and, thereby, cure the illness. The healer returned the patient and the object to a proper balance or relationship.

The healer believed he communicated with and appeased the spirits through his invocations. Some healers made cuts in the body to let blood or pus run out—to encourage the evil spirit to leave. Sacrifices or offerings were often made to the gods to abate their anger. In very early times, it was the voice of the healer and his accepted, even magical, powers that were valued even above those of the natural substances that accompanied the ritual.

That nonmedicinal approaches worked attests to the power of suggestion that can mobilize processes in our own body and help relieve symptoms. Today, we call this the "placebo effect"—the relief of disease or symptoms caused by the mere suggestion that the medication will work and that the person will get better. The "placebo effect" is that force or reaction that influences disease via changes in the body in response to positive feelings about treatment. In testing the efficacy of a drug, contemporary clinical researchers always give a placebo, usually a sugar or chalk pill, to half the patients in the test while the other half receives the real medication. Even the doctors giving out the drug do not know which pill they are dispensing. If the drug shows a statistically higher benefit over the placebo, then it is considered truly therapeutic. It has demonstrated its potency. While yet to be fully understood, the placebo effect may be linked to products that the cells of our bodies make in response to certain stimuli, such as positive suggestion.

In time, new discoveries led to changes in therapeutic approach. As they were found effective, they were passed on to future generations as part of oral tradition and later written. In the 3500-year-old Egyptian papyri and the 3000-year-old Babylonian cuneiform tablets, we find evidence that a multitude of different natural products were mixed into pumice or potion to treat illnesses. In general, the role ascribed to these medicinals was to drive out the "demons" that had invaded the bodies. In the tradition of their predecessors, healers believed, by and large, that it was still the "soul" of an herb that appeased the "soul" of an offended spirit. In one ancient account, a physician–priest directed his colleagues to combine a medicinal herb, which assuaged the soul, with some bitter substance, generally a form of animal dung, to drive evil spirits away. Such inventive potions served to reinforce the overriding faith in verbal appeals directed to spirits. Even today, while modern medicine no longer attributes disease to evil spirits, people still accept bitterness in certain preparations, believing in its enhanced ability to cure. Perhaps the sense of sacrifice or pain must accompany the treatment in order for the medicine to work.

The earliest written documents, from the 16th to 17th centuries B.C., present details of pathology and diseases, as well as of treatments. In one Egyptian papyrus, discovered by George Ebers in 1872–73, we find complete descriptions of medications used in 1552 B.C., a time when Moses was only 21 years old. They probably represent medicinal preparations that had been passed down to subsequent generations for a thousand or more years. These prescriptions were apparently prepared by an ancestral precursor to our modern pharmacist. The preparations, while hardly like any we use today, represented remedies that had been found to abate disease symptoms. They included whole parts of plants and animals, living and dead. Generally, a special chant accompanied the medication. Verbal appeal was an important component of the therapy.

For diarrhea, the ancient Egyptians suggested a mixture of figs, grapes, sycamore fruit, gum, and yellow ochre—along with a special chant. For headache, "skull of silicrus fish is boiled with oil and the head is rubbed therewith for four days."[1]

The cuneiform tablet writings of ancient Assyria, dating from over 2500 years ago, also document the mixture of healing substances:[2]

- For a headache, the following direction was given. "Thou shalt beat up fennel in cow's milk or cow's urine, wash his head (therewith), reduce *barhus*, bray (it) press it on his head, annoint with oil . . ."

- For an eye problem this advice was given. "Thou shalt disembowel a yellow frog, mix its gall in curd, apply to the eyes."
- For toothache, people were advised, "Thou shalt slit a leek, rub on the root of the tooth and he shall recover."

These writings highlight the extent of medicinals known and used and the importance placed on their proper preparations and applications.

The prescription of medicinals to the afflicted was not uniformly accepted. As Greek mythology relates, Aesculapius angered the gods by taking the ability to cure disease away from them and giving it to mankind. Aesculapius, regarded by most as an ancient physician and by some as a deity, reportedly made house calls to visit his patients in bed. From writings of this time, we can deduce that he probably used emetics and purgatives, incisions, and ointments. When his medicines failed, he relied on his faith in music and incantations to heal. His disciples, advocates of medicines, were seen as enemies of the traditional priesthood, which believed its members had exclusive power over disease. According to them, offerings should be made not to the patient, but to the holy shrines. The Aesculapians, however, who were priests as well as physicians, developed their own religious following and temples. Their delivery of medicinals directly to the ill person clearly defined the movement away from purely spiritual appeal to tangible cures, residing in organic materials found in natural sources.

During a large part of our later recorded history, sickness was attributed to having too much or too little of necessary bodily substances. Ancient Greeks defined illness as the imbalance of four body humors—blood, phlegm, yellow bile, and black bile—that embodied a mixture of four universal qualities: moist, dry, cold, and warm. Hippocrates, and later Aristotle in the 4th century B.C., articulated this fundamental concept in their teachings.

In disease, something either had to be replaced or had to be removed in order to restore health. Influenced by this interpretation, medical practitioners often removed humors; hence, the practice of using leeches attached to the body to suck blood. Under the guidance of this theory, physicians tested and found other effective, natural substances. We know today that these substances, such as plant leaves and roots, contained active chemical ingredients, including antibiotics, that were the agents responsible for the relief of symptoms and cure of the disease. The treatments became classified according to their abilities to correct disturbances in the body, such as fever, rapid heart beat, and muscle weakness.

These ideas formed the rationale for a more organized approach to disease introduced in the second century by a Greek physician named Galen (130–200 A.D.), who is perhaps history's most influential doctor (Figure 3.1). His more than 22 volumes of teachings greatly influenced medicine and attracted followers for more than 14 centuries. It was Galen who first showed that blood, not air, flowed through arteries. He also proved that urine came from the kidneys. But his fame came from his approach to healing, which led to the discovery and use of other substances as medicinals. Galen based his medical theories and ideas on how natural products found in their native surroundings fit the particular needs of the body as defined by the "humors." Believing "contraria contrarius curantum," or "that which is opposite cures," he was led to try interesting, new substances. Galen chose an item because it appeared to represent one of the four universal qualities making up the human temperament and gave it to patients based on its ability to restore what he considered absent or off balance. For instance, vinegar was recommended for the burning heart. He borrowed from the old Greek writings, widely from Hippocrates, and added much more of his own scholarship. Some estimate that he more than doubled the medical literature of the time.

The "galenicals" he gathered were simple organic or mineral ingredients. No substance was outside the realm of potential use—the bark of trees, the juices of berries or algae found in

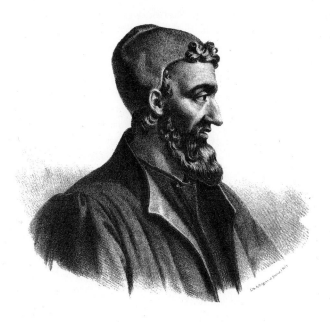

Figure 3.1 Claude Galen (130–200 A.D.) prepared and used natural substances as medicinals based on their presumed ability to correct an imbalance in the body's humors. Galen chose substances that were opposite in quality to the body humor that he believed was out of balance. His influence on medical therapeutics lasted more than one thousand years. (Rare books section, Countway Medical Library, Boston.)

still waters. Galen's preparations were, by their very essence, hard to standardize but were more understandable and more directed to particular disease symptoms than those prominent in the years preceding him. Some were prepared by Galen and his followers and given to the patient; others were made by the patients themselves on advice of the Galenist physicians. No details on amounts were provided. Galen let each patient or physician decide. By consequence, during this extended period of Galen's influence, drug-making by pharmaceutical professionals, who were beginning to surface, progressed very slowly.

Although viewed as separate entities, medicine (the science of diagnosis and treatment) and pharmacy (the science of drug production and drug activity) evolved alongside each other. Certain early physicians devoted their energies to both. Aristotle carried his own medicines with him and had them available to give directly to his patients. To a large extent, so did Galen and his followers. But the pharmacist emerged where his expertise was needed, particularly with the demand for defined medicinal substances. In the 13th and 14th centuries in England and Germany, apothecary shops appeared and a real separation of physician and pharmacist took place. With the establishment of the pharmacist and the apothecary, attention was increasingly focused on the disease and its symptoms.

Consumer confidence and quality control of the product became important early on. In the 13th century, Frederick II, emperor of Spain and Italy, issued an edict that required every medical man to give information against any pharmacist who sold "bad" medicine:

> Every physician given a license to practice must take an oath that he shall faithfully fulfill all the requirements of the law, and in addition, whenever it comes to his knowledge that any apothecary has for sale drugs that are of less than normal strength, he shall report him to the court. . . .[3]

He went on to disallow any physician from owning an apothecary himself, a desirable mandate not practiced in parts of the world today. The Emperor saw clearly how a conflict of interest could emerge.

Today we obtain our medications from pharmacies, generally through the prescription of a physician. The pharmacy represents, therefore, the physical provider of medication and also assures its quality. The two professionals, doctor and pharmacist, are thus intertwined in the delivery of medicine to the patient. In certain countries and for certain drugs, however, medicines can be obtained without a doctor's prescription, that is, as an over-the-counter item. This practice, which we shall discuss further, has broken the tie between these two professions, permitting and encouraging self-medication.

Galen's influence extended into the 16th century. Then Paracelsus, the son of a country physician from Basel, introduced methods for extracting the active components. Not readily accepted by his peers because of his flamboyant style and ideas, he argued for understanding the essence of medical treatment. He simplified and gave uniformity to Galen's prescriptions. But he took a vastly different approach from the established Galenical method. He treated the diseased organ, not the symptom. He discarded the concept of the "humors." In fact, he publicly burned the works of Galen.

In contrast to Galen, who chose medicinals that represented the opposite of the disease symptoms, Paracelsus believed in the doctrine of "signatures" or "similars." Thus, the flower or the leaf of a plant that most closely resembled the diseased organ was often selected to heal the organ. Historians tell us that the discovery of digitalis, the single most important drug used to treat heart disease today, came from the ancient, traditional use of the extract of the heart-shaped foxglove leaf to treat symptoms then that we now know were related to the heart.

Instead of Galen's ill-defined proportions, Paracelsus and followers described exact amounts of particular ingredients to be used. More than ever before, the pharmacy began to find its role in society. This novel approach, however, was not accepted universally, and, throughout the 17th century, followers of Paracelsus remained in conflict with the Galenists.

The therapeutics of the Middle Ages and Renaissance continued to be a mixture of superstition from ancient times and experimental daring of the great physicians of the day. Potions, strange mixtures concocted for good and evil intent and used throughout recorded ancient civilization, continued in use into the Middle Ages. As Shakespeare reminded us in the witches' song in his play *Macbeth* (Act IV, Scene 1):

Fillet of a fenny snake
In the caldron boil and bake
Eye of newt and toe of frog
Wool of bat and tongue of dog
Adders' fork and blindworm's sting
Lizard's leg and howlet's wing
For a charm of powerful trouble
Like a Hell broth boil and bubble.

Belief that disease is caused by evil spirits held sway. Into the 18th century, people wore purple amulets around their necks to ward off the plague and other diseases. They contained bits of frog, other animals, and the ever-potent animal dung. Often extracts of human skulls taken from dead bodies were part of these preparations. Exorcisms, used to drive out altered disease states in the human body, continued into the late 1800s.

But the times were being primed for the appearance of "modern" medicines, that is, those bottled and sold as preparations to relieve health problems. Throughout the 17th and 18th centuries, various medicines became commonly available for a variety of ailments. Some from England were imported to the United States. Advertisements for these medications filled almanacs in the United States and England. As early as 1685, Samuel Atkins carried this advertisement in his first almanac:

> Some experienced medicines, sold by William Bradford at Philadelphia. Charles Marshall's Spiritus Mundus, being an excellent medicine against all sorts of Fevers and Agues, Surfeits, Gripes, Pleurisies, etc. A present remedy for the Gravel and Stone, which seldom fails to give ease in half an hour.[4]

The practice continued into the 18th century. Nathaniel Whittimore from Boston offered in 1721, "Sundry very excellent medicines found out to cure both hot and cold gouts, dropsies, consumptions, perilous coughs, fevers, ague and most other diseases incident to Mankind . . . To be had at a reasonable price, of N. Whittemore."[4]

These advertisements for over-the-counter medications epito-

mize the already prevalent trend toward self-treatment. This was
further realized in whole books devoted to self-medication. To
some extent these books fulfilled a real need; they also played on
people's search for easy cures. One book by John Theobald first
appeared in 1764 and was already in a third edition by the end
of the same year (Figure 3.2). In it, Theobald put together a

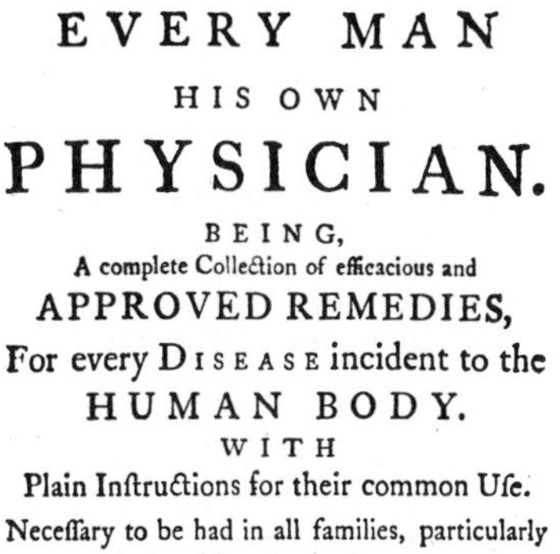

EVERY MAN

HIS OWN

PHYSICIAN.

BEING,

A complete Collection of efficacious and

APPROVED REMEDIES,

For every DISEASE incident to the

HUMAN BODY.

WITH

Plain Inftructions for their common Ufe.

Neceffary to be had in all families, particularly
thofe refiding in the Country.

By JOHN THEOBALD, M. D.

Author of MEDULLA MEDICINÆ.

Compiled at the command of his Royal
Highnefs the Duke of CUMBERLAND.

*Difeafes are cured, not by eloquence, but by remedies, fo that
if a perfon without any learning be well acquainted with
thofe remedies that have been difcovered by practice, he
will be a much greater phyfician than one who has culti-
vated his talent in fpeaking without experience.*

CELSUS.

The THIRD EDITION, with great
ADDITIONS and IMPROVEMENETS.

LONDON:

Printed and fold by W. GRIFFIN, in FETTER-LANE.

MDCCLXIV.

[Price Eighteen-pence.]

Figure 3.2 Almanacs of this kind were popular in the 17th century and into the
18th century. Many books published in England were sold in the United States.
These books formalized "home remedies" and propagated self-medication (Rare
books section, Countway Medical Library, Boston).

compendium of remedies that he had collected from different sources. He explained that "these receipts are published chiefly for the use of persons residing in the country whose convenience or abilities will not allow of the attendance of a physician or apothecary."[5]

The ingredients of these remedies were in part galenicals but had the details of a modern pharmaceutical preparation. For instance, one such home remedy for pleurisy states, "Bleed frequently till the pain abates, apply a blister to the side, and take half a pint of the following infusion twice a day: take fresh horse-dung six ounces and pour on it a pint of boiling Pennyroyal water, strain it when cold and add a quarter of an ounce of Venice treacle, mix for use."[5] Theobold credited this remedy to the London physician John Quincy, who published a list of dispensaries during the early part of the 18th century.

It can be argued that these books and almanacs may have offered benefits to some, in terms of easy harmless "home remedies," but they opened up opportunities for quackery, playing on people's wishes to find a ready cure for their ailments. Most pertinent to present-day antibiotic misuse, however, was the encouragement for self-medication. This practice, prominent today, has potentially harmful effects not only on the individual, but in the case of antibiotics, on the sustained efficacy of these drugs. While present-day societies have reaped the rewards of past discovery, they have also inherited a potentially harmful relaxed attitude toward medications, particularly evident in regard to antibiotics.

A significant development in understanding disease appeared in the 19th century and led to yet another change in the direction of drug discovery. Although the concept of a diseased state of man, rather than a causal agent, was still in vogue, as we noted earlier, Louis Pasteur, working and writing in Paris at the time, produced convincing observations that "êtres vivants," "living creatures" or microorganisms, were causing human disease (Figure 3.3). Linking these microscopic beings to disease was a major step into the modern era of medicine. With the "germ" as a

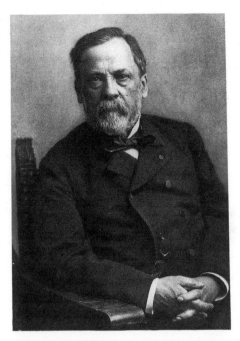

Figure 3.3   Louis Pasteur (1822–1895), the French chemist responsible for success-fully arguing the "germ theory of disease," revolutionized our view of infectious diseases and of the approach to therapy (Rare books section, Countway Medical Library, Boston).

causative agent, the scene was set for tremendous advancement in the field of medical science.

This framework encouraged scientists to look for drugs as defined therapeutic entities directed to fight bacteria. The ability of these agents to kill bacteria and cure previously fatal diseases was nothing less than a miracle. Their discovery satisfied the never-ending appeal of miraculous curing agents able to restore well-being to the patient and to society.

The mindset of the individuals looking for new drugs and the attitude of the public toward medicines have shaped historical developments of medicine and in turn antibiotics. Self-medication and the ready availability of medical products has played into the present-day attitude that antibiotics are cure-alls. A naive confidence that antibiotic use is only beneficial has led to misuse and overuse and the consequent selection of mutant forms of bacteria resistant to their killing effects.

Chapter 4

ANTIBIOTIC RESISTANCE

Microbial Adaptation and Evolution

Today most bacteria that were previously universally susceptible to antibiotics are resistant to at least some antibiotics and, in some cases, to many different ones. We must face this unsettling situation now, only 100 years since the recognition that bacteria cause disease and only 50 years since the discovery of antibiotics. When antibiotics came into being, they were a godsend. Natural substances made by one microorganism could inhibit growth and kill another. Scientists learned to produce, harvest, and purify these substances for treatment of diseases caused by microorganisms. The dramatic effect of antibiotics in treating previously fatal diseases led to enormous expectations. Even minor symptoms, once left to our own body defenses, were given over to drug therapy, in many cases to these new "miracle" agents. But there was an unexpected consequence to this reliance on antibiotics. Bacteria developed ways to resist them. With increased and prolonged use came selection of bacteria that were no longer killed by the antibiotic. These strains propagated and took their places in the environment, coming back to cause infections that were not cured by these drugs.

How did bacteria "learn" to withstand the onslaught of antibiotics? The answer has revealed an unexpected panoply of genes and transferable genetic elements that exist in bacteria and endow their bacterial hosts with resistance mechanisms.

BACTERIAL PLASMIDS

Bacteria, like all living beings, must be able to cope with and even adapt to changing environments in order to survive. The traits encoded by genes in the DNA of their single chromosome are often not enough to ensure their survival in the face of adverse conditions. Therefore, bacteria, through evolution, have acquired and maintained supplemental genetic information in the form of accessory pieces of DNA that are separate from the chromosome itself. These so-called "plasmids" exist as independent self-duplicating genetic elements—like minichromosomes—carrying as few as three and as many as 300 different additional genes. Anywhere from one to as many as a thousand copies of a plasmid may exist in a cell. Many different plasmids can reside in the same cell. The information that the plasmids carry enables bacteria to perform new functions and engender new products that are not part of their chromosomal genetic repertoires (Figure 4.1).

The traits borne by plasmids are numerous and versatile. They enable bacteria to adhere to the cells lining the human gastrointestinal tract so that these bacteria can withstand the continuous flow of food residues passing through it. They help their host bacterium survive a sudden change in the environment, such as extremes of temperature. Unlike the physical and physiological changes that occur in trees and plants with seasons, or that occur in animals that hibernate during winter, these plasmid-

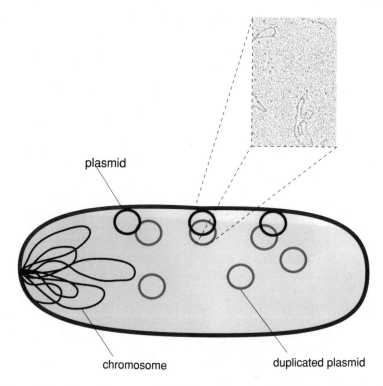

plasmid

chromosome   duplicated plasmid

Figure 4.1. Plasmids are small, circular pieces of self-replicating, double-stranded DNA that are accessory genetic elements in the cell. There may be as few as one or as many as a thousand copies in a cell. They provide other traits not specified by the cell's single chromosome. The inset is an electron micrograph of a plasmid (18,480-fold magnification) isolated from *Escherichia coli* (Bonnie Marshall, Tufts University School of Medicine).

borne "survival" traits are there to be called into play at any time. Thus, bacteria bearing accessory traits can better accommodate the sludge of sewage systems, the fast moving waters of rivers and streams, the rise and fall of temperatures, the killing effects of ultraviolet light from the sun, and the changing humidity of soils.

But perhaps the most important function of plasmids in bacteria that we confront today is their ability to help their bacterial hosts resist being killed by antibiotics. Not all plasmids bear all the traits discussed above, including the genes for antibiotic resistance, but the numbers that do bear resistance traits are increasing, as we shall see later.

Plasmids, like bacterial viruses, multiply within bacteria. They are visible only by the electron microscope, being more than a million-fold smaller than bacteria (Figure 4.1). Unlike viruses, plasmids lack a protective outer protein coat and, therefore, cannot survive outside the bacterial cell. They have no chance of multiplying except in the cell and are, thus, dependent on the cell. In one sense, although they are not independent microorganisms, they exist as a kind of parasite of the cell. Their very presence illustrates the evolution of a mutually helpful relationship between these genetic elements and bacteria. Since their destiny rests entirely with the host bacterium, they cannot afford to kill this host. Thus, viruses and plasmids are guided by a different rationale in their continued existence. The plasmid, like the faithful servant, depends on its host and, in return, protects the life of its host by providing needed survival traits. The virus, like a Trojan horse, gets through the host wall barrier, and, once inside, goes on to kill the host cell when multiplying its progeny. A virus can afford to be more selfish than a plasmid since it can survive as an entity apart from the cell; however, it too must get into a cell in order to make copies of itself.

Plasmids are not static elements. They are constantly subject to change by either losing or acquiring new genes. Two plasmids in the same bacterial cell can combine to form one large plasmid or to exchange pieces of their DNA. Often these exchanges involve genes for antibiotic resistance. Thus, a single bacterium can acquire multiple antibiotic resistance genes on its favorite plasmid. By exchanging and picking up different genes, one extrachromosomal element can emerge with the ability to provide its host with traits for wide environmental survival, not only new ways to get nutrients but also new ways to prevent being killed.

EMERGENCE OF RESISTANCE PLASMIDS

Soon after the introduction of penicillin into clinical medicine, bacteria insensitive to the antibiotic appeared. Initially, and for many years afterwards, these penicillin-resistant bacteria were found in the hospitals where most of the penicillin was being used. Resistant hospital strains were different from the mutant strains that scientists had already isolated in the laboratory. Whereas the laboratory bacterial mutants were resistant to relatively small amounts of penicillin by being less permeable to the drug, the resistant strains that emerged in hospital patients were resistant to large concentrations of the drug. The reason was that hospital strains had acquired a plasmid that enabled the cell to destroy penicillin. Increasing the quantity of penicillin did not help because these resistant bacteria were able to destroy large amounts of the antibiotic. These unexpected findings produced a sobering effect on the optimism that followed the discovery of penicillin. They showed that bacteria had developed a way to protect themselves in a totally unforeseen way. Plasmids, whose existence was virtually unknown until resistance was uncovered, posed quite a threat to the therapeutic miracles that penicillin had brought. Once their presence was noted, their impact on public health soon became realized as patients failed to get better despite penicillin therapy.

DISCOVERY OF TRANSFERABLE RESISTANCE

Our knowledge of the existence of transferable antibiotic resistance plasmids is relatively new and came more than ten years after the discovery of pencillin-resistant staphylococci. In 1959, a bacterial dysentery plaguing numbers of patients in Japan was linked to the bacterium *Shigella dysenteriae*. What was unique about this bacterium was not the disease it caused, but its capacity to resist four different kinds of antibacterial agents available at that time, namely tetracycline, sulfonamide, streptomycin and chloramphenicol. Multiple drug resistance had been almost unheard of at the time. Of interest, however, in 1955 before this epidemic, a *S. dysenteriae* with similar resistances was isolated from a Japanese woman on her return from Hong Kong. Since no one else was involved, little was made of the observation then.

The 1959 event held more surprises. *Escherichia coli*, normal intestinal bacteria found in the same diarrhea specimens, were also found to be resistant to the *same* four drugs. Not only had scientists discovered a combination of multiple antibiotic resistances not previously seen, but for the first time it was appearing in two different kinds of bacteria. This was an alarming revelation and the Japanese scientists knew it.

Let us return to penicillin resistance. When it appeared in bacteria, the resistance gene specified the production of an enzyme that destroyed penicillin. This resistance enzyme affected only penicillin; it did not touch sulfonamides, the only other antibacterial agents then in use. Based on what was known about mutants at the time, this resistance could have been the result of a mutation on the bacterial chromosome. Later it was shown to reside on a plasmid. In the case of these multiresistant *Shigella*, it was difficult to even imagine single mutations as the basis for resistance to four different drugs. Each mutation occurs rarely, only once in every 10 million to 100 million multiplications of bacteria. By extrapolating from standard mutation rates, Japanese scientists realized that the resistance to four different kinds of antibiotics in a single microorganism would have required a seemingly unattainable frequency of chromosome mutations. Even if each mutation occurred once in 10 million, mutations to four drugs would have needed 10 million $\times$ 10 million $\times$ 10 million $\times$ 10 million or 10^{28} doublings! This realization led the astute Japanese workers to look for a different genetic basis for multiple drug resistance. They guessed that the resistance traits might be associated with genes *not* on the chromosome. Evidence for "extrachromosomal" genes had emerged a decade before when Joshua Lederberg and Edward Tatum, working together, described sexual exchange in *E. coli*. Traits in one bacterium could be transferred to another if the two had contact. Later the phenomenon was linked to the transfer of extrachromosomal sex factors, called fertility or "F" factors. They and others soon reported that bacteria bearing these F factors could exchange genes on their chromosomes. Occasionally some of the chromosomal genes remained associated with the F factors.

The finding of the same four resistances in two different kinds of bacteria from the same diarrhea specimen provided the impetus for scientists to look for an F factorlike transfer. It did indeed exist. Like F factors, the transferable elements were also plasmids. They were called "R" (resistance) factors to distinguish them from F factors. Unlike F factors, whose transfer was limited to a very small group of related bacteria, multiple resistance was transferable among a wide number of bacterial types. Furthermore, it was revealed that R factors carried genes and traits not normally found on the chromosome, that is, they came from other bacterial hosts.

The discovery of R factors was both exciting and worrisome. Their existence implied that resistances could be carried in the relatively harmless gut bacterium *E. coli* and could be transferred to other bacterial species harmful to man, such as the *Shigella dysenteriae* that caused dysentery in the Japanese patients. In one area, 60% of *Shigella* isolated were resistant, of which no fewer than 90% were multidrug resistant. Another bacterial family that could accept these plasmids was the *Salmonellae*, whose members cause diarrhea, blood and bone infections, and typhoid fever.

Soon after, reports of transferable plasmids bearing multiple drug resistance came from England, Germany, the United States, and elsewhere. By 1966, more than half of about 300 *E. coli* strains from feces and urine of patients at the Pretoria Hospital in South Africa showed resistance to one or more of the antibacterial drugs. At the same time, almost 25% of *Salmonella* strains isolated in a Boston hospital were multidrug resistant and carried R factors. This phenomenon was not occurring just in Japan—it was happening worldwide.

This discovery of transferable R factors, thirty years ago,

opened the eyes of microbiologists and medical scientists to a breadth of gene spread never before imagined. Transfer of resistance genes could occur among bacterial species more genetically and evolutionarily distant than a horse is from a cow. Though not fully realized at the time, these findings predicted the widespread nature of antibiotic resistance we face today.

ORIGINS OF RESISTANCE GENES: IMPACT OF ANTIBIOTICS

Genes for resistance are not new creations. We now know that they appeared, albeit in low frequency, in environmental bacterial species long before they entered bacteria that cause human diseases. Many kinds of bacteria carry resistance plasmids, which very likely protect them from the killing effects of antibiotics and other naturally occurring substances. After all, penicillin and other antibiotics are produced in nature by microorganisms. Some data suggest that resistance genes evolved from genes found in the very microorganisms that produce antibiotics—the soil bacteria. This would be a likely place for them to reside in order to protect these antibiotic producers from their own killing products. We can speculate that resistance genes somehow escaped from soil microorganisms and, after passage and evolution in other bacteria, have entered those that have direct contact with humans.

A number of studies revealed that resistance genes existed before the development and clinical use of antibiotics. In a mid-1960s study of the feces from 47 Kalahari bushmen who had no known contact with other people or with antibiotics, as well as fecal samples from over 300 wild animals in South Africa and Rhodesia (now Zimbabwe), low but detectable numbers of resistant bacteria were found. None of the resistances were transferable. Other studies in "antibiotic-virgin" areas also showed resistant genes in bacteria and these transferred to other bacteria.

One 1969 study examined the frequency of R factors in the

intestinal flora of people living in the bush of the Solomon Islands, where antibiotics had not been introduced. Soil bacteria were also studied. Among 40 isolates, two—one from soil and one an *E. coli* from a native living there—contained resistant bacteria bearing transferable R factors. At about the same time, studies in a community in north Borneo, where antibiotics had not been used, also revealed the presence of antibiotic-resistant *E. coli* bearing transferable resistance. In all studies, although they were not common, resistant bacteria gave a clear message—the resistance genes were *not* newly created by the use of antibiotics. They were already present where antibiotics had never been introduced.

While human usage of antibiotics did not somehow *create* antibiotic resistance genes, it certainly has contributed to the increase in their numbers and the numbers of resistant bacteria. By introducing large quantities of these drugs into the environment, we have drastically altered the ecology of microbes. We have unwittingly given a selective advantage to resistant bacteria.

Today, everywhere, we see the results of the widespread massive use of antibiotics. Under antibiotic selective pressure, resistant strains have emerged "victorious" in the world of microbial competition. In certain parts of the world, antibiotic resistant strains of common bacteria have edged out those susceptible to antibiotics. But the advantage given to resistant bacteria is evident only if an antibiotic is present. Otherwise, resistant and susceptible bacteria are indistinguishable by size, color, growth, and reproductive ability. The prior existence of resistance genes in nature explains why they could appear relatively soon after antibiotics became therapeutic agents. The finding illustrates how nature continues to move toward a balance by imbuing the wily bacteria with the means to survive and persist despite scientists' persistent attempts to destroy them.

Antibiotic usage has stimulated evolutionary changes that are unparalleled in recorded biologic history. Prior records and studies of bacteria did not suggest they were undergoing evolution more quickly than were other living beings. But artificial selection by man-made drugs has fostered changes that are moving at an extremely rapid pace. During these almost five decades of antibiotic use, common bacteria have appeared with combinations of genes coding for resistance to multiple antibiotics; some are resistant to eight to ten *different* drugs. This phenomenon has occurred through the joining together of different and even rarely found resistance genes onto common plasmids. Geneticists, fascinated by their appearances, and clinicians, awed by their consequences, are moved to try to understand just how these genetic elements were created and maintained.

ORIGIN OF PLASMIDS

The discovery of plasmids as the genetic vehicles of resistance genes raised questions about their origins. Were plasmids a recent creation, like a new disease, or did they exist before, perhaps in a different environment?

Naomi Datta and colleagues at the Royal Postgraduate Medical School in London examined over 300 different clinical specimens of *E. coli* and other intestinal bacteria that had been isolated from humans and stored during the period 1917 to 1954. Most of the specimens predated any major clinical use of antibiotics. None of the isolated specimens bore a transferable resistance. The only resistance found was in a microorganism naturally resistant to tetracycline. More importantly, the scientists showed that this strain collection contained plasmids—the same kinds of plasmids we see today—only *none bore antibiotic resistance genes*. This finding concurred with the examination of fecal samples from the Kalahari bushmen and animals in South Africa, where larger numbers of bacteria still showed low frequency of resistant bacteria.

An investigation from our laboratory in Boston in the early 1980s addressed this same question about plasmid origins in another natural environment. We examined the levels of resistance in the gut bacteria of nonhuman primates, namely baboons living without human contact in the wild savannah of Amboseli National Park in Kenya. Our on-site investigator, Rosalind Rolland, a second-year Tufts University veterinary student, flew to Kenya with boxes of disposable plates, pipettes, flasks, and powdered nutrients—all the supplies required for the three-month field project. Before 4 o'clock each morning, she crawled out of her tent into the Land Rover. She and a team of Cornell anthropologists led by Glenn Hausfater drove 40 kilometers into the wild brush of the national reserve (Figure 4.2). Feces from about 50 baboons were collected and studied soon after they were excreted. The behavioral sociologists knew each animal by name and family ties, so each fecal sample could be assigned to a particular baboon. In this way, single samples from each baboon were examined and members of the same baboon family were compared. The investigators found only low levels of resistant bacteria in the fecal samples. Some of the resistances were on transferable plasmids. Of interest,

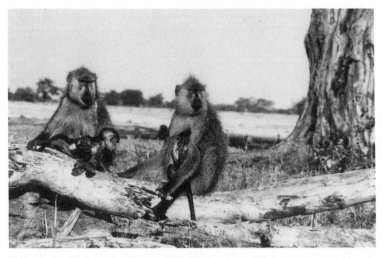

Figure 4.2.   Baboons (*Papio cynocephalus*) in their natural habitat in a national park in Kenya. The fecal flora from these wild animals had little, if any, antibiotic resistance.

the few resistant strains identified appeared in the intestinal flora of members of the same baboon family.

These and other studies substantiate that resistance genes are not new, nor are plasmids. They have been around for a long time.

GENE EXCHANGE: CONJUGATION, TRANSPOSITION, TRANSDUCTION, AND TRANSFORMATION

The process by which bacteria share genetic material is as intricate and surprising as the fact that it occurs at all. In one kind of bacterial mating called "conjugation," a fascinating but not fully understood event occurs. First, the bacterial cell bearing the plasmid produces a fine filamentous protein structure called a "pilus," which reaches out to another bacterium. Upon contact, the pilus draws the two bacteria together. Then the "donor" bacterium makes a duplicate of its plasmid and passes its plasmids (there can be more than one) to the other cell. Both cells now carry a copy of the resistance plasmid (Figure 4.3). The event causes the creation of both a new resistant strain and a new donor. As transfers continue, new and old donors find new recipients and an exponential increase in resistant strains occurs. The transfer process requires such specialized mating apparati, consisting of ten to fifteen different proteins, that scientists believe these proteins have evolved solely for the purpose of the genetic exchanges. Gene transfer must be integral and critical to the overall survival of bacteria, providing a way for bacteria to adapt to difficult conditions. It is a means of producing great diversity and enormous genetic flexibility in the face of changing environmental threats. One survivor can produce new copies of itself, as well as recruit new resistant neighbors.

There is even more complexity and breadth to gene exchange. Small plasmids, which cannot direct their own transfer, "ride" into a new bacterium "on the backs" of larger plasmids. As before,

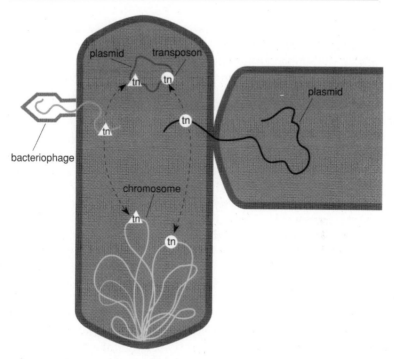

Figure 4.3. Conjugation via plasmids, transposition via transposons (tn), and transduction via phages are common means by which genetic material flows from one bacterial cell to another. Transfer of genes takes place among bacteria of all types (Bonnie Marshall, Tufts University School of Medicine).

it is the duplicate plasmid that moves. Ensuing events can further favor the spread of the plasmid copies or its genes. For example, if the new host contains a resident plasmid that can transfer itself, these small plasmids can use it to move into yet other kinds of bacteria. Once in these new hosts, plasmids can spread further. Plasmids entering new types of bacteria can move with their new hosts to environments not visited before. So we see the same kinds of plasmids in bacteria inhabiting the intestinal tracts of humans, as well as those of animals. The same plasmids are found in marine bacteria and soil bacteria. Sometimes, however, the plasmid can find a hostile environment within its new host. In this case, it does not get duplicated, and, therefore, is not donated to new progeny. Thus, it is lost when the original host dies.

Perhaps one of the largest geographic spreads of a plasmid was documented recently. Thomas O'Brien and his associates of the Brigham and Women's Hospital in Boston noted a similarity in a multiresistance plasmid from one of their hospital patients and one reported five years earlier from Seattle, Washington. After genetic sleuthing, these investigators showed that this same plasmid, in different bacterial hosts, had made its way into nine different states and even as far as Caracas, Venezuela. This was intercontinental spread on what they called an "epidemic plasmid."

Other bacteria, notably the enterococci, which we mentioned before, have evolved another kind of mating system. These bacteria secrete substances called pheromones, attractants, which cause two different cells, often called "mating types," to clump together. While closely attached, the two bacteria exchange whole plasmids or pieces of them (Figure 4.4). This aggregation presumably causes a fusion of the cell membranes and an unimpeded free exchange of elements inside the cell, including the plasmid bearing its genes. Streptococci and staphylococci also produce sex pheromones that attract other bacteria of the same or even different types. The resemblance of this microbial mating system to that of other life forms is remarkable. Living creatures as diverse as insects, goldfish, and birds reportedly attract opposite mating types by producing pheromones. Even men and women release pheromones, body scents, that attract the opposite sex.

Resistance transfer may occur in other ways. We are learning that bacteria exchange genes without the need for their plasmids to remain in the new cell. This is possible because the resistance gene (or genes) resides on yet smaller pieces of DNA, called "transposons," which can jump from one piece of DNA, such as a plasmid, or chromosome to another and vice versa (see Figure 4.3).

Transposons would do well on a Darwinian scale—they have

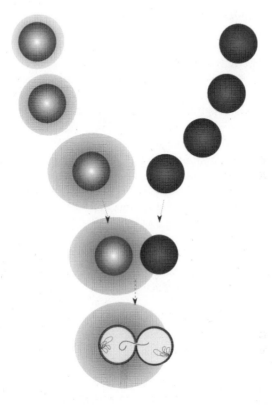

Figure 4.4. Pheromone-induced genetic exchange among enterococci is another way by which plasmids and genes are exchanged. The donor (left) produces a substance, a pheromone, which draws another bacterium (right) to it. Once together, a genetic exchange takes place. This form of transfer appears in other Gram-positive bacteria as well, such as *Staphylococcus* (Bonnie Marshall, Tufts University School of Medicine).

strong survival potential. Unlike plasmids, they do not rely on a particular host cell or any particular host DNA molecule in order to exist or multiply. Transposons easily become part of diverse microbial species because they "jump ship" onto the host chromosome or onto a resident plasmid already stably docked in the cell. For instance, a plasmid can enter *E. coli* from *Hemophilus influenzae* and deliver its resistance gene, but cannot survive itself. It does not find a place to hitch up. The transposon has another option. It can jump onto the new host chromosome or onto a resident plasmid. While the new host may lose the plasmid and even its copy, the transposon with its resistance information will remain with the new cell since it has found a stable place in the new host. In an analogous way, the common pneumococcus, which causes lobar pneumonia, exchanges resistance genes that are on its chromosome with other streptococci. They do so by moving transposons, called "conjugal transposons," into the new cell.

Another way that bacteria can transfer genes, both from plasmids and from their chromosomes, is via bacterial viruses, called bacteriophages. Phages, as they are more commonly known, infect only those bacterial hosts that have a particular membrane site to which they can attach. Once there, the phage injects its DNA into the cell. The transferred DNA has two choices: it can multiply rapidly and kill the cell; or it can find a place to sit on the chromosome. If it chooses the chromosome, it may carry pieces of the host chromosome with it when it later pops out of the chromosome to make its progeny. Thus, when the phage multiplies, the chromosomal piece does also and follows the fate of the phage. Upon entering a second host, the phage delivers itself as well as this "carried along" piece of DNA from its previous host. Gene exchange takes place when the phage and its chromosomal DNA piece integrate into the second host's chromosome. Another way that a phage can transfer genes is via transposons. If the phage has picked up a transposon, it will deliver the transposon to the new host when it injects its DNA. Afterward, the transposon can follow the same route as the phage, or, as it does with plasmids, the transposon can jump off the phage and place itself into a resident plasmid or onto the chromosome of the new host bacterial cell.

Gene transfer can also occur via naked DNA itself. The process, called transformation, involves the pickup by a recipient bacterium of pieces of free DNA released by another bacterium. Once taken up, the DNA can become part of the DNA of the recipient cell.

Thus, through many different, but often integrative, transfer processes, pieces of DNA, genes, can move from one bacterial cell to another, including bacteria of very different types.

GENE EXCHANGES IN NATURE

We now know that bacteria exchange genes readily in nature. Antibiotic resistance has allowed us to see just how extensive these transfers can be, because resistance genes are so easy to identify and follow. By plating on an agar plate containing an antibiotic, investigators can identify strains that are resistant to that drug. By placing antibiotic-impregnated discs on a plate spread with the strain and incubated, scientists can learn how many resistances are present in the strain. More recently, with the advent of gene cloning, each resistance gene can be identified as a special gene, not just as a resistance trait. This is done by a method called DNA:DNA hybridization. One biochemically or radio-actively marked strand of DNA of the gene being followed is asked to find its copy, a second strand, on a filter paper bearing DNA from the resistant strains of interest. If a match is there, the marked strand will join to the DNA on the paper. A "hybridiza-tion" occurs, which can be noted by the radioactive or biochemical signal. In this way, the exact gene can be tracked among different strains resistant to the same drug.

The hybridization method has shown that antibiotic resis-tance genes, formerly found among a narrow group of bacteria, are present in different kinds of bacteria residing in very different places. It appears that previously susceptible bacterial types have "picked up" the resistance genes during some kind of contact with resistant bacteria. Resistance genes initially identified in Gram-positive bacteria were found in Gram-negative bacteria. These kinds of bacteria had not previously been known to exchange genetic material.

For instance, one type of gene, *tet*(M), which specifies tetracycline resistance (there are more than a dozen different types), was initially found in enterococci, intestinal bacteria of humans and other animals. The gene was soon recognized in other very different bacterial species that cause diseases of the respiratory and urinary tracts. Marilyn Roberts and her group at the University of Washington have tracked by DNA:DNA hybridization this resistance gene to bacteria frequenting different ecological niches and bearing very different cell wall structures.

Let's imagine that different bacteria find themselves confronted by an area saturated with tetracycline. In order to enter and survive, they must become resistant to the drug. The survivors are those that received the resistance gene from a donor before going in. The others die or escape elsewhere (Figure 4.5). Today, *tet*(M) has been picked up by pathogens and nonpathogens alike, all resistant to tetracyclines. Many nonpathogens living in the urogenital or respiratory tracts bear the gene. Although they are no trouble to us, they become reservoirs of the gene and potential "donors" to new pathogens entering the scene. The microbial reservoirs include both aerobic and anaerobic bacteria, many of which were never before known to exchange genes. The *tet*(M) example has revolutionized our view of "wide" when we speak of widespread microbial spread of resistance genes.

Staphylococci with the penicillinase gene have been around for the last 50 years—having appeared during the first uses of penicillin. Until recently, the gene seemed confined to this type of bacteria. Then, Barbara Murray and colleagues in Texas found that enterococci, intestinal bacteria that we have discussed before, began to break down penicillins for the first time. In fact, this ability further thwarted antibiotic treatment. Surprisingly, after

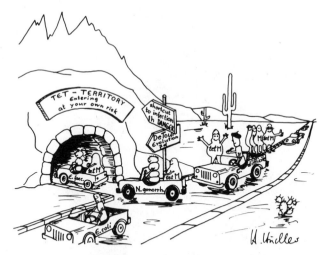

Figure 4.5. Tetracycline resistance specified by the *tet*(M) resistance determinant is common in bacteria associated with humans, especially in bacteria in the respiratory and urogenital tracts. The high frequency of the gene suggests that donors are plentiful and recipients are all too eager to obtain this lifesaving resistance determinant (Herbert Hächler, University of Zurich, Zurich, Switzerland).

DNA:DNA hybridizations were performed, they found that the new gene in the enterococcus was not original—it was the old gene from staphylococcus, having found its way into a new host. It took almost 50 years for this apparent transfer to take place. The gene is not an exact copy but has some subtle changes that may have made it acceptable in the enterococcus. The penicillinase gene is present on multiresistance plasmids that are transferable among other enterococci. Such an event is troubling since such a transferable gene would certainly wreak medical havoc if passed to the Group A streptococci, a group of Gram-positive bacteria that causes "strep throat" and "scarlet fever." So far, these bacteria are extremely unusual among Gram-positive cocci in that they are still sensitive to penicillins.

Some form of transposonlike transfer is the possible route of

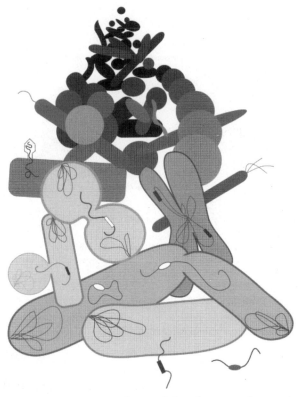

Figure 4.6. Bacteria are not single populations but part of a vast interactive microbial world exchanging plasmids and genes allowing adaptation to changing environments (Bonnie Marshall, Tufts University School of Medicine).

entry of the staphylococcal penicillinase gene into enterococci. Such is also the presumed route by which the ampicillin resistance gene came into *Hemophilus influenzae*. This gene, first noted in the 1960s, was later shown to reside on a transposon on plasmids in *Escherichia coli* and other gut bacteria. Not until the mid 1970s was the same resistance gene and part of the transposon found unexpectedly on plasmids in resistant strains of *H. influenzae*. The plasmids in *Hemophilus* were not those found in *E. coli*—only the resistance transposon was the same. A similar process begins to explain how the same ampicillin resistance transposon appeared in the very different bacterial species, *Neisseria gonorrhoeae*, that causes the venereal disease gonorrhea. It made *Neisseria* resistant to penicillin. Once again, the resistance gene was the same as initially found in *E. coli*, only now it was on a plasmid found commonly in *Neisseria*. Since there are common plasmids found in *N. gonorrhoeae* and *H. influenzae*, we cannot be sure if the transposon jumped onto the plasmid in *Neisseria* and then went to *Hemophilus* or vice versa. Alternatively, it could have happened independently in both species. Scientists are still trying to discover the actual pathway of this exchange. What is clear, however, is that such diverse exchanges can and do take place.

Today, we know that genes bearing different traits, originally considered confined to certain bacterial types that share similarity of shape or cell wall, are now found among bacteria of very different sizes, shapes, and colors. These include rodlike and spherelike bacteria and those that grow with or without air. While these exchanges may be rare events, there do not appear to be conditions that prohibit such exchanges from occurring if potential donors and recipients are given appropriate circumstances for such an exchange. This seeming dissolution of boundaries between categories of bacteria has completely changed scientists' views of microbiology. One begins to see bacteria, not as individual species, but as a vast array of interacting constituents of an integrated microbial world (Figure 4.6).

NONTRANSFERABLE RESISTANCES: STILL A PROBLEM

Resistance may be spread even if it is not on a transferable element. Strains of bacteria are appearing resistant to the new quinolone group of antimicrobials such as norfloxacin, ofloxacin, and ciprofloxacin. These drugs are used for an increasing number of infections, including urinary tract, intestinal, and bone infections. Resistance, when it appears, is specified by genes naturally present on the cell's chromosome but not normally active, that is, they are not expressing the protein product. At a certain frequency, the bacteria sustain a spontaneous mutation that allows expression of this resistance gene. If the quinolones are present, these resistant forms survive and propagate.

Fortunately, so far, none of the quinolone resistance traits have emerged on transferable elements. Therefore, the resistance problem is with the host bacterium and efforts can be directed at it, with less concern about spread of the gene to neighboring bacteria. While this latter feature may offer some confinement of the resistance trait, we are learning that the new resistant hosts themselves are sufficiently mobile that they are spreading globally and at an increasing frequency. Most notable are the multiresistant *Staphylococcus aureus* strains, which have added chromosomal quinolone resistance to their plasmid, transposon, and other resistance genes. *E. coli* and *Pseudomonas* are also appearing with quinolone resistance at unexpectedly high frequencies.

Rifampin resistance also results from a mutation on the bacterial chromosome. This drug is used for ear infections, resistant skin infections, and tuberculosis. Today, a major problem in the treatment of tuberculosis is the appearance of a resistant tubercle bacillus that does not respond to rifampin, isoniazid, and other agents previously successful in curing this disease. And these mutants confront public health officials in countries worldwide. Thus, while these resistances are not on transferable elements, their appearance in this disease-causing bacterium has created a major deterrent to cure and a major world health problem. We shall discuss later the devastating impact of these multidrug resistant bacteria in New York City.

Methicillin, as we discussed earlier, was synthesized to treat staphylococci that produced the penicillin-degrading enzyme, β-lactamase. Being insensitive to the enzyme, methicillin seemed a clear winner. But to everyone's dismay, methicillin-resistant mutants appeared, first in northern Europe and now worldwide. Again, this resistance gene is on the cell chromosome, making its host cell wall insensitive to the drug and rendering it useless against disease.

Another chromosomally located resistance determinant is one that specifies destruction of cephalosporin-type antibiotics. These cephalosporinase genes are located on the chromosomes of certain Gram-negative bacteria. Generally, these enzymes are produced in very small amounts and so the microorganisms appear to be sensitive to the cephalosporins. Once treatment with one of these cephalosporins begins, however, a small but significant fraction of cells shows an increase in production of the inactivating enzyme. By this means, the microorganism becomes fully resistant. The increasing use of the newer, so-called "third-generation" cephalosporins, together with this potential resistance gene, has caused *Enterobacter* to become the third leading cause of hospital infections caused by Gram-negative bacteria today.

In one study involving multiple medical centers that looked at the kinds of bacteria isolated from the bloodstreams of hospital patients, those patients receiving a third-generation cephalosporin were three times more likely to have multidrug-resistant *Enterobacter* as the causative agent than those who did not receive the cephalosporin. Moreover, those patients in whom *Enterobacter* were found had a twofold higher chance of dying from the disease than those who had an antibiotic-susceptible one. Thus, by an uncommon chromosomal trait, an uncommon pathogen has now become very prominent in hospital infections. The study's authors suggest that "more judicious use of third-generation cephalosporins" may decrease the incidence of these hospital infections and also the mortality from them.

DIVERSE MECHANISMS FOR RESISTANCE

Bacteria have acquired fascinating and novel ways to survive antibiotics. Some do not let the antibiotic in or export it out;

others chemically modify the antibiotic so it is no longer active; others simply destroy it; and still others replace a sensitive antibiotic target with one that is insensitive to the drug. We shall briefly discuss each of these kinds of mechanisms.

Decreased Drug Entry

In order for antibiotics to work, they must penetrate the cell. Many do so by making use of transport systems already in the bacteria. Thus, in a suicidal fashion, bacteria furnish special transport systems for some growth-inhibiting substances and supply their own routes for death. For this reason, transport into the cell was one of the resistance mechanisms expected in resistant bacteria and was the mechanism for penicillin resistance first seen in the laboratory mutants produced by Alexander Fleming. But resistance by this mechanism is generally not very powerful since the block in uptake is not great and can often be overcome by giving more of the drug. Decreased permeability, however, when

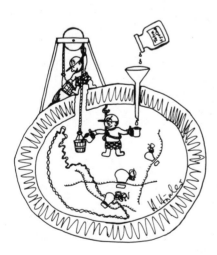

Figure 4.7. One mechanism for tetracycline resistance involves actively pumping the drug out of the cell, keeping it away from its active target, the ribosome (Herbert Hächler, University of Zurich, Zurich, Switzerland).

accompanying other mechanisms of resistance, can provide the host with very high levels of resistance that are insurmountable by increased antibiotic dosage.

Another, more potent, way to prevent uptake of an antibiotic into the bacterial cell is to increase its export from the cell. This is how many tetracycline resistant bacteria survive. By a unique mechanism, the resistant cell pumps tetracycline out of the cell faster than it can accumulate inside (Figure 4.7). This pump is made of a protein produced in the cell by the tetracycline resistance gene. In order to work, it requires energy from the cell. The efflux of tetracycline is very efficient, allowing resistant cells to survive up to 100 times the therapeutic dose of tetracycline. Active efflux as a mechanism for bacterial drug resistance has also been found for other antibiotics, such as erythromycin, and other toxic elements, such as heavy metals.

Inactivation of the Antibiotic

In contrast to the way the resistant cell deals with tetracycline, many other resistance mechanisms are dependent on specific destructive or modifying enzymes that defuse the power of the antibiotic. Such enzymes have amazed investigators, not only by their specificity for a particular drug, but also by the broad variety of destructive and modifying enzymes that exist for the same antibiotic. Under the direction of the resistance genes, cells destroy penicillins by penicillinases and cephalosporins by cephalosporinases. There are more than two dozen different kinds of penicillin/cephalosporin-inactivating enzymes specified by different resistance genes. The enzymes can be distinguished by their sizes and by their abilities to inactivate different types of penicillins and cephalosporins.

Enzymes alter, and so inactivate, streptomycin, kanamycin, and other drugs of the structurally related "aminoglycoside" group by placing a chemical residue on the drug. The modified drug has trouble getting into the cell and, therefore, cannot bind to the cell's protein synthesizing machinery, the ribosomes, where it normally inhibits protein synthesis. Similarly, resistance to chloramphenicol is also mediated by an enzyme that modifies and so destroys the drug's activity.

Alteration in the Antibiotic Target

Instead of acting on the antibiotic itself, other mechanisms affect the target of the antibiotic's action in the bacterium. This is one way that bacteria become resistant to the new quinolones and to rifampin, drugs we discussed earlier. By a cell mutation, the enzyme (on which either quinolones or rifampin acts) changes, making the cell insensitive to that antibiotic.

In a similar fashion but by a different mechanism, the erythromycin resistance gene, usually carried on plasmids, leads to a change in the ribosome, the site of action of erythromycin. The modification does not affect the ability of this important cellular structure to make proteins, but does eliminate its binding site for the antibiotic. A second kind of mechanism for tetracycline resistance, specified by the *tet*(M) gene, also works by somehow altering its target, the ribosome. A protein product of this tetracycline resistance gene appears to "protect" the ribosome from the inhibitory action of tetracycline by keeping the drug away from its target (Figure 4.8).

Substitution of Antibiotic-Insensitive Targets

Resistance to trimethoprim and the sulfonamides also involves a mechanism that leaves these synthetic antimicrobials unchanged. Normally, the antimicrobials act by inhibiting key enzymes needed for reproducing the chromosome of the bacterial cell. In resistant bacteria, the drug is not altered, nor is the host bacterium changed. Instead the resistant cell produces another enzyme "copy," like the one the bacteria need and the one on which the antimicrobial acts, only this new one is not inhibited

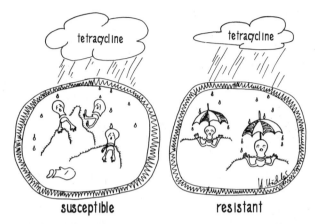

Figure 4.8. A second mechanism for tetracycline resistance shields the ribosome from tetracycline, thus preventing the drug from inhibiting protein synthesis (Herbert Hächler, University of Zurich, Zurich, Switzerland).

by the drug. In the presence of trimethoprim-insensitive or sulfonamide-insensitive enzymes, the cell survives contact with these growth-inhibitory drugs.

In view of the discovery that there are naturally occurring resistance genes able to deal with these synthetic antibacterial agents, we must rethink our idea that resistance genes were created and sustained in bacteria in order to protect them from antibiotics. While this may still be true in some cases, quite possibly resistance genes have other purposes and have merely been selected by the antibiotics we use because they "happen" to allow the bacterial host to resist the drug. Once so selected and present in the environment, however, use of these drugs will augment the frequency of resistance genes. And this is exactly what happens.

In one study in the mid-1980s, American students entering Mexico for the first time were placed on the drug combination trimethoprim/sulfamethoxazole as prophylaxis for diarrhea during their two-week stay. This practice is not generally accepted today. In any case, over this time period, the intestinal bacterial flora of students taking the drug were compared with the bacteria of those who were not. There was a rapid appearance of intestinal *E. coli* bearing transferable resistance to both of the drugs in those students taking the antibiotic combination. While these "new" *E. coli* were no health problem to the students, their appearance illustrated the high frequency of these resistance genes already in the Mexican environment at that time and the selective effect of the drugs being taken.

In a study completed in 1987, almost 10% of first year students at a Boston medical school were found to harbor *E. coli* resistant to this drug combination at a level of 10% or more of the total *E. coli* in their gastrointestinal tracts. The students had no contact with patients and had not been taking any antibiotics for at least a month.

The trimethoprim/sulfamethoxazole combination was introduced in the 1970s. Studies show that in less than one generation of clinical use of this combination, resistant strains had reached levels easily detected in our resident bacterial flora. Normally such resistant *E. coli* would cause no problem, but they serve as reservoirs of these resistance genes. Sometimes even *E. coli* can give trouble. Two leukemia patients in Los Angeles died from bloodstream infections caused by just such a trimethoprim/sulfamethoxazole resistant *E. coli* that was, until that time, totally unexpected.

RESISTANCE MECHANISMS AND THE ENVIRONMENT

Because the actions of resistant bacteria do not destroy the tetracyclines, macrolides, trimethoprim, sulfonamides, and the quinolones, these antibiotics can remain intact in the environment unless destroyed by high temperatures or other physical damage, such as ultraviolet light from the sun. As active antibiotics, they continue to kill off susceptible bacteria with which they have contact and select surviving resistant forms. The resistant strains have an advantage and become more numerous. Thus, these kinds of resistance mechanisms, unlike the penicillinases, serve only the bacteria that bear them. On the other hand, if resistant bacteria are using mechanisms that inactivate the antibiotic, such as penicillinases, they will remove the antibiotic from the environment. This effect will remove continued selection of resistant strains and protect sensitive bacteria that happen to be in their vicinity. From the medical standpoint, this can be a problem. For instance, a penicillin-susceptible pathogen may be difficult to eradicate in the throat if a penicillinase-producing strain is also there. The β-lactamase producer protects the susceptible pathogen by destroying the penicillin.

From the environmental viewpoint, however, degradative proteins are helpful. They remove the active drug from the environment and, therefore, reduce its ability to select for resistant strains. Herein lies another facet of the antibiotic paradox—resistance mechanisms, like the antibiotics themselves, can play both positive (for the environment) and negative (for the patient) roles.

MULTIPLE-DRUG RESISTANCE

Single drug resistance can occur via a chromosomal mutation that generally limits drug entry into the cell or alters the target site of the antibiotic. These kinds of "simple" mutants rarely create a medical problem, since we usually have many alternative active antibiotics from which to choose. Today, we are confounded by the phenomenon of *multiple*-drug resistance and the existence of separate determinants of resistance on plasmids and transposons. Multidrug resistance is the *rule*, not the exception, among resistant bacteria. To some extent, this situation has occurred through the sequential acquisition of each resistance trait following the use of the selecting antibiotic. The first antibiotic began by selecting a single resistance gene. Eventually, however, bacteria resistant to the first antibiotic picked up resistances to others as they were introduced into the environment. The bacteria, however, did not lose the previously acquired resistance traits. It's like a snowball rolling downhill, picking up snow and any debris during its transit, becoming bigger in the process and not losing what it had acquired before (Figure 4.9). So do plasmids as they "roll" through the environment.

A fascinating correlation was revealed by Jacob Kupersztoch of Mexico, who now teaches at the University of Texas in Dallas. He recorded the predominant types of multiresistant *Shigella* present in Mexico. He found that the resistant *Shigella* reflected the chronology of different antibiotics being introduced into the

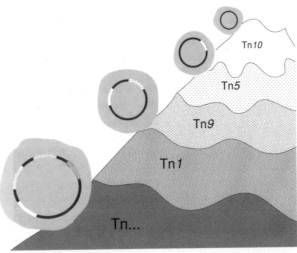

Figure 4.9. Plasmids pick up resistance genes on transposons as they move through the environment. By retaining previous ones and picking up new ones, they increase in size, like a snowball rolling down a hill (Bonnie Marshall, Tufts University School of Medicine).

country. The most common resistances were to the drugs first introduced in the 1940s, the sulfonamides, followed by those introduced later: penicillin, chloramphenicol, and tetracycline. A similar phenomenon was noted *during* an epidemic of cholera in Tanzania in the mid-1970s. As doctors seized on new drugs, the infecting *Vibrio cholerae* appeared with resistance to each subsequently used antibiotic. Scientists see transposons as responsible for this process, using plasmids as their vehicles for insertion, duplication, and transfer.

Given enough antibiotic use and its consequent selection of resistant strains, resistance increases and rears a foreboding and Hydralike head. Thus, with time, we see the creation of microorganisms resistant, not to just one drug, but to multiple drugs. It is the multiply resistant bacteria appearing in different diseases and ecologic settings that truly threaten our ability to treat infections successfully today.

One of the most difficult present-day problems of multidrug resistance is facing public health authorities in New York City—tuberculosis resistant to multiple drugs. Individuals infected with these resistant bacteria have died, despite attempted therapy. The emergence of resistance in the microorganisms is considered the result of patients' not completing a normal course of therapy, inappropriate treatments, and antibiotic misuse. The resistant strains first gained prominence when prison inmates died. The problem was also being recognized in intravenous drug users, as well as the indigent and homeless populations. Following the New York City outbreak, two other hospitals in New York State reported the problem. At least eight healthcare workers have contracted the disease. There is anticipatory concern of wider spread. For instance, among tuberculosis patients nationwide, most are infected with the AIDS virus, of which many now bear resistant strains of TB.

The incidence of tuberculosis began to increase in the United States at the end of the 1970s, even before AIDS appeared on the scene. From this time onward, many TB health programs had their budgets drastically cut or their programs discontinued. The timing of these events was bad. Although resistance was reported periodically, it had never reached dangerous proportions until the present situation. Now, drastic measures are needed. Attention is directed both at finding appropriate therapy for these resistant strains and for preventing their spread. Recent meetings have been held in order to alert clinicians and raise awareness of the problem. More than $1 million were given to research and work in New York City alone. The interest now is a far cry from what it has been. Suddenly, "TB is out of control in this country," as one official remarked at a recent meeting. Multidrug resistance in this microorganism has created truly one of the most critical medical emergencies of the present decade.

The pneumococci represent another current ongoing multi-drug-resistant problem. In Eastern Europe, Central America, Spain, South Africa, and elsewhere, this microorganism, the cause of infection of one or more of the lobes of the lung, called lobar (pneumococcal) pneumonia, has appeared with resistance to penicillin, erythromycin, and tetracycline as well as trimethoprim/sulfamethoxazole—all first-line drugs for therapy. The result has been a high rate of treatment failures and search for alternative modes. The choices are slim when the microorganisms are so multiresistant.

Multiple resistance in *Shigella* has been an obstacle to therapy of dysentery in Africa and other developing nations for many years. But the problem has emerged in the United States as well. The Centers for Disease Control recently reported outbreaks of multiply resistant *Shigella* among native Americans on Hopi and Navajo reservations in Arizona. Of concern was the resistance to trimethoprim, an agent previously effective against multidrug-resistant strains. Farther away, but at about the same time, Bulgaria reported resistance to four to six drugs, including trimethoprim in *Shigella*. And, among over 3000 isolates of resistant *Shigella* in Vietnam, 90% were insensitive to three or more antibiotics. These findings show the worldwide nature of this multiresistance phenomenon. Without the use of these previously effective drugs, these countries must use more costly newer ones, assuming they are even affordable and available.

Multidrug resistance in *Staphylococcus aureus* ravaged hospital patients in Melbourne, Australia, in the 1980s before public health measures and one antibiotic came to the rescue. We shall discuss this key incident and its ramifications later.

SINGLE ANTIBIOTIC USE LEADS TO MULTIDRUG RESISTANCE

For reasons beyond our present understanding, the continuous use of even a single antibiotic over a period of weeks to months will select bacteria with resistance to different kinds of antibiotics, in addition to the one in use. This multiple resistance is not linked to a single gene or a single mechanism. The phenomenon is again linked to plasmids collecting different transposons. It is easy to understand the selection of multidrug resistance if plasmids already bear more than one resistance determinant. The phenomenon we are addressing, however, is the gradual appearance of more and more resistance in the same bacteria with time on the *single* antibiotic. This seeming recruitment of multiple resistance transposons under selection by a single antibiotic is very curious.

Why should bacteria want or need to resist more than the drug with which they are being confronted? The phenomenon has been observed repeatedly. For instance, female patients being treated with only tetracycline for urinary tract infections were found to excrete, in their feces, *E. coli* with more and more different kinds of resistances as the therapy extended into weeks. The same findings were observed in patients taking tetracycline for treatment of acne. As weeks went by, more and more bacteria in their guts became resistant to as many as four to six different antibiotics.

Besides bacteria in the gut, those on the skin have also responded to this chronic use of a single antibiotic. Wesley Kloos from North Carolina State University examined the susceptibility of different kinds of staphylococci on the skin of patients taking either tetracycline or erythromycin continuously on a weekly basis for acne. He showed the gradual transition with time from antibiotic susceptible types to those with multiple resistance. Other studies of humans and animals have substantiated the reproducibility of this phenomenon. It usually takes two weeks or more on the antibiotic for the multiresistance to appear. The reason that this recruitment of multiple resistance occurs is still unclear, although the players involved, namely transposons and plasmids, are well known.

Recently, members of my research group discovered that this evolution of multidrug resistance will occur even in the absence of plasmids and transposons. While growing a plasmid-free *E. coli* in the isolated environment of a test tube in the presence of small amounts of tetracycline, we obtained bacteria surviving the treatment. Quite unexpectedly, on further study, the same surviving bacteria showed resistance to seven other different antibiotics as well. This phenomenon occurred repeatedly with other *E. coli* isolated from feces of different people or from animal feces. Yet these bacteria had no plasmids and no resistance transposons.

With increasing antibiotic contact, the initial mutants emerged with higher and higher levels of resistance. The initial mutation that led to multiresistance has been located in a single site on the *E. coli* chromosome. Many genes on the chromosome are needed to produce all these different resistances, but all are under the control of this single, mutated chromosomal site. Even more surprising, the resistances were not limited to naturally occurring antibiotics, but also the newer synthetic antimicrobials, the quinolones, such as norfloxacin and ciprofloxacin. This same multiple resistance locus has been found on the chromosomes of other types of bacteria, thus enlarging the kinds of bacteria potentially subject to this form of mutation to multidrug resistance.

These environmental and test-tube studies show that bacteria must have some intrinsic, yet unexplained, reason for displaying multiple resistance when confronted with a single drug. It is almost as if bacteria strategically anticipate the confrontation of other drugs when they resist one. If resistance genes are present in the environment, as on transposons and plasmids, the surviving bacteria recruit these genes, thereby acquiring immediate high-level resistance. Otherwise, they still have a chromosomal mutation that provides low-level protection and survival of at least some of the cell population.

MULTIRESISTANCE: A GENERAL BIOLOGICAL PHENOMENON

Multidrug resistance is not unique to bacteria but occurs in other microorganisms, including insects, infectious parasites, and human cancer cells (Figure 4.10). Agricultural farmers are faced with destructive insects resistant and multiresistant to pesticides. Malaria was initially controlled by attacking the mosquito, carrier of the malarial parasite, with DDT. Today the resurgence of malaria can be explained by the appearance of mosquitos that not only have resistance to DDT but that also carry resistance to other insecticides as well.

In a large part of the world, the malaria parasite itself has become resistant to chloroquine as well as to other drugs used to treat malaria patients. Today, this multidrug resistance has become a leading obstacle to curing the disease and protecting against infection.

Treatment of human cancers with one growth-inhibiting drug can lead to the emergence of small numbers of surviving cells that bear resistance to that drug as well as to other structurally different chemotherapeutic agents. Here, as in the mutated *E. coli* and in the malaria parasite, the trait for these resistances already existed in silent form on the chromosomes of the cell but mutated to overt expression. Tumors consist of cancer cells with different levels of

WINSTON-SALEM JOURNAL

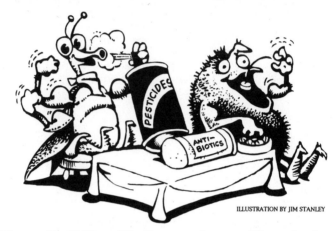

ILLUSTRATION BY JIM STANLEY

Bugs Building Up Immunity to Chemicals

Figure 4.10. Multidrug resistance is common to bacteria and parasites, linked to overuse of growth-inhibiting agents. This cartoon was inspired by a symposium in Chicago in 1987 at the annual meeting of the American Association for Advancement of Science. Scientists shared data that revealed a resistance problem among different living organisms. (Illustration by Jim Stanley, *Winston-Salem Journal*, Winston-Salem, North Carolina.)

susceptibility to the anticancer drugs. When a patient is treated, those tumor cells with slightly less susceptibility, that is, those that are slightly resistant, become dominant in the tumor because the drugs select and kill off the drug-sensitive tumor cells that competed with the resistant mutants for blood supply. As with bacterial infections, these resistant cells multiply and become the dominant entity in the tumor. The cancer no longer responds to the therapy. Today, multidrug resistance is a phenomenon that thwarts our ability to cure cancer, perversely mimicking the problem with bacteria.

BACTERIAL RESISTANCE: A PROBLEM AFFECTING DECISION-MAKING

Bacterial resistance to antibiotics is not a new creation of the past 40 years. It has, however, become a new clinical problem, because preexistent, naturally occurring plasmids have become equipped with previously rare resistance genes. The combination of resistance genes on transferable plasmids has enhanced spread of resistance.Bacteria have demonstrated to us a remarkable fluidity in their genetic material. Under the threat of antibiotics, a small number of them can achieve a tenacious survival mode, either by chromosomal mutation, or more frequently, by acquisition of new genes. These events allow them to persist and grow in the direct path of what had been efficient killing agents, the antibiotics. We now find increased numbers and types of resistant strains, along with new combinations of resistances in even one bacterium. All of this has appeared within the short time span of two generations. We are presently witnessing a massive, unprecedented, evolutionary change in bacteria. By developing and using antibiotics, we have, in a sense, caused these events to spiral. We are at a new era of understanding—considerations regarding bacterial resistance must be part of our decision-making and part of our planning for the future of antibiotic therapy.

Chapter 5

THE ANTIBIOTIC MYTH

Antibiotics continue to be our major therapeutic resource for curing and preventing infectious diseases. Their introduction in the 1940s totally revolutionized the treatment of human infections, and the successes of antibiotics continue to prompt their immediate use when an infectious bacterial cause is suspected. The myth of the so-called "miracle drugs" persists today, however, as people unthinkingly demand antibiotics for ailments for which these agents have no value. In turn, their effectiveness is often diminished, tarnishing their reputations and putting us at risk from unresponding infection by drug resistant forms of bacteria.

HUMAN USE AND ABUSE

A look at several examples of people and instances where antibiotics have been misused can be illuminating.

Ms. E., an attractive, bright, 25-year-old lawyer fresh from law school landed a job in one of the well-known 100-member New York City law firms. She had just finished her first set of briefs for one of the senior partners. She was proud of her work and satisfied with her position, but long hours and little sleep had gradually taken their toll. "I must be coming down with a cold," she told the secretary as she walked out wearily that day, suffering from a scratchy throat, achy muscles, and a mild headache. "I hope I'll be in tomorrow, but I'll see." At home she prepared hot soup and tea but relief was only temporary. She had joined a Community Health Plan and decided to make use of it the next day.

"But there's nothing seriously wrong," Dr. R. told her. "It's just a virus. You have no fever. Your throat is red but hardly inflamed. I suggest you get some rest. Take some aspirin. I've taken a throat culture and done a test here in my office. It's negative for the streptococcus that causes 'strep throat.' I seriously doubt that you have anything other than a cold for which you do not need a prescription. The generalized achiness tells me that you've got one of the flu viruses."

"But I need an antibiotic, Doctor," Ms. E. insisted. "I've always gotten an antibiotic before when I've had a cold and it has always helped me."

"Well, that may appear to be the case," replied the doctor. "But if you had symptoms like these, you had a common cold caused by a virus. You would have gotten better without the antibiotic. That's what you have now and antibiotics are not my recommendation."

Ms. E. was not satisfied and, in fact, found herself another physician in the area and got her antibiotic. She changed her Health Plan. "I can't afford to be sick," she told me. "How do you doctors know that an antibiotic would not help *me*?"

Ms. E., like many young adults, has been brought up on the "antibiotics-work-for-a-cold" myth. In fact, the cold virus is not touched by antibiotics. The French have a wonderful saying that portrays this ineffectiveness: "An untreated cold goes on for seven days; a treated cold lasts a week."

Despite physicians' advice to the contrary, a person searching long enough will eventually find a physician who will prescribe an antibiotic, even when one is not indicated. Success in the search may be influenced by how well the patient knows the physician and the risk that denial of the drug might lead to the physician's losing the patient. To some extent this casual attitude about antibiotics is due to ignorance on both sides, the consumer and the prescriber. The consumer, believing in the miracle drug, knows nothing about the potential harm in taking an antibiotic in a trivial fashion. The physician, worried about losing the patient, may rationalize that a bacterium may be involved but, if pushed, will probably admit that he or she thinks it is likely just a viral cold. Of course, there may also be a tiny minority of physicians who still believe in the powers of antibiotics in all instances.

*   *   *   *   *

In another setting, a less subjective factor can influence the patient's ability to obtain the antibiotic. Who is paying for the drug? In the private sector this usually means the patient, and if the patient is willing to buy the medication and the doctor provides the prescription, the antibiotic is obtained. In a prepaid health program, the result may be different. The program foots the bill. The doctors may be less apt to give in to patient demand and patients have less say in the matter. There is no risk to the physician of losing the person as a patient and, in fact, physician prescribing practice is often monitored. Antibiotics and other drugs are generally under closer scrutiny in these instances than in the totally private sector. Although a prepaid program's goal is to provide the best care to the patient, there is a concerted effort to keep costs down. Here there is often an ongoing bureaucratic assessment of the rationale for prescriptions, which does not prevail in the private outpatient arena.

In many parts of the world, such as Mexico, the Caribbean, South America, and Southeast Asia, antibiotics can be obtained directly from physicians or over-the-counter in pharmacies. This setting precludes the need to "plead" or "argue" for the drug. Over-the-counter availability generates and propagates a "laissez-faire" attitude toward medicines that leads to antibiotic misuse. On a visit to Santiago, Chile to discuss the problem of antibiotic misuse, I stayed at a hotel that happened to be across the street from a pharmacy. Curious, I went over to see how easy it would be to obtain an antibiotic. In the store window were bottles of a number of different antibiotics, all available to the consumer. To my surprise, there was a sale going on. For that week, and only that week, I could get the locally made chloramphenicol for 30% off the list price. If I wanted the American-made product, I could still get a 10% discount (Figure 5.1). While this may seem shock-

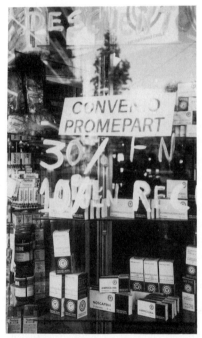

Figure 5.1.   The over-the-counter sale of antibiotics in pharmacies is a common occurrence in Central and South America and other countries of the developing world. During this particular week in Santiago, Chile there was a sale (DES-CUENTO) on chloramphenicol with 30% off the locally produced product or 10% off the imported product. Other antibiotics were also displayed in the windows and readily available to the consumer.

ing, it is even more disturbing that a potentially hazardous antibiotic should be dispensed so freely.

In these same countries, limited supplies of many drugs are provided to government clinics to be used for treating the vast majority of people in those countries. When in short supply, antibiotics are prescribed in small amounts so as to reserve them for those in real need. Insufficient supplies dictate shorter periods of treatment and smaller dosages. Herein lies another aspect of the problem. Short courses of therapy, using less of the antibiotic, may not totally cure the disease. In some instances, only the first day's treatment of the antibiotic may be offered to the patient, leaving the rest to be bought at the local pharmacy. This can pose a severe burden to the patient for whom a day's antibiotic can equal a day's pay. Inadequate treatment leads to continued illness and potential spread of the infectious bacteria to other members of the community.

*   *   *   *   *

While the poor get inadequate amounts of antibiotic, the wealthy in these countries can easily obtain any of these drugs they want. A case in point is Mr. C., a respected 49-year-old businessman from Buenos Aires, who had accumulated millions from his family fortune and from his personal investments. He was the father of five young children and the husband of a lovely 40-year-old woman, a former model in Buenos Aires. An energetic man, he spent more than two-thirds of his day pursuing business ventures but still found time to spend with his family. Mr. C. did not like to be held back by sore throats and mild cold symptoms. While he maintained great faith in the advice and medications given to him by his family physician, he generally treated himself with readily available drugs that he bought at the local pharmacy. On one occasion, however, Mr. C. had had an exceptionally bad cough and fever, on and off for several weeks. He had trouble starting his day because of extreme fatigue. During that time he had been taking several different antibiotics that he had obtained from his pharmacy, to no avail.

Dr. S. noticed an unusual pallor that he had not recognized in

Mr. C.'s previous visits over the last ten years. "I think we should get a blood test on you," he said. "I've also noticed some tiny red spots coming up on my legs and arms," Mr. C. added. Dr. S. examined the areas and recognized them as tiny bleeds in the skin. He suspected a serious disease. He looked up and asked, "What kinds of drugs have you gotten your hands on? Did you take any chloramphenicol?" Dr. S. was concerned about a critical side effect of this antibiotic—its ability to shut down blood production in the bone marrow and even cause leukemia. "No, not that I'm aware of. I keep a number of these drugs at home, but I don't remember that one," Mr. C. answered.

The blood test on Mr. C. showed him to be anemic, evidenced by a reduction in circulating red cells. His white count was elevated; he had very few platelets, the blood components that help to control bleeding. It was this problem that led to the red marks on his skin. The white cells themselves appeared abnormal. Dr. S. diagnosed acute leukemia.

Mr. C. was flown to a medical center in Boston where the diagnosis was confirmed. He had a high fever, and his white cell count had climbed to 20 times the normal number and consisted mostly of abnormal-looking white cells. The hematology team put him on a ten-day course of chemotherapeutic drugs and warned that he would become very weak. While the drugs were given to rid his body of all the leukemic cells, each day of therapy brought on worse symptoms. He became nauseated and had to be treated with antinausea drugs. Additionally, he needed antibiotics to treat his infection.

In one arm went the drugs for his leukemia and in the other arm went the high-powered antibiotics for the infection. For some reason, however, the fever did not abate. The intern told Mr. C. that an intestinal bacterium, *Escherichia coli*, was circulating in his bloodstream. What the intern did not share with him was that this particular *E. coli* had proven resistant to *eight* different antibiotics.

Both the intern and the resident had never seen this severe a resistance problem before. A normal *E. coli* should be killed by any of the antibiotics, including ampicillin, tetracycline, cephalosporins, gentamicin, and other members of the aminoglycoside family of antibiotics. Mr. C.'s microorganism was resistant to these and to other penicillins, as well as other highly potent antibiotics. Even the newer members of the cephalosporin family of anti-biotics proved ineffective. Later, physicians determined that the resistances were to many of the drugs that Mr. C. had been taking freely over the last ten years. This microorganism had accumu-lated resistance not only to these, but to a vast array of other effective drugs carried on the same plasmid.

Over the ten-day course of chemotherapy, the bone marrow was rid of all detectable leukemic cells. On the 17th day, the bone marrow test showed that Mr. C. had come through the chemo-therapy as well as any other patient so treated and should be on his way to an initial remission. But fever and infection persisted. The high doses of antibiotics were not controlling the infection and were troublesome because of their possible interference with the blood's ability to clot. His platelet count was critically low as well. On day 20, with no warning, while speaking to his nurse, his eyes turned upward and he began to shake. He suddenly lost consciousness. When he woke up several hours later he could not talk. He had apparently sustained a bleed in his head. His blood still lacked normal white cells and his body was still ravaged by the multi-resistant *E. coli*. Over the next two days, he went further downhill. And on the 22nd day after chemotherapy, with his bone marrow free of detectable leukemia, Mr. C. died of bleeding and overwhelming infection. An autopsy showed that the resistant *E. coli* had produced multiple sites of infection in his liver and other organs.

Although Mr. C.'s leukemia was responding to treatment, his infection was out of control. He succumbed to infection, *not* to leukemia. The cause was a microorganism brought with him into the hospital—one found in his own intestinal tract, the probable result of his own repeated antibiotic usage. Other far-reaching potential consequences of this resistance are troubling and unde-niable. Resistant strains selected in one person can move to infect other people. The appearance of this unusual multiply resistant strain of bacteria, "imported" so to speak, could lead to its spread to other hospital patients. Additionally, the genes specifying the multiple resistance could be exchanged among other bacteria native to this new environment. These new recipient bacterial types could associate with other people and even cause disease. Intermittent and repeated antibiotic use, as illustrated in this patient, creates an environment not only of microorganisms resistant to the drug being used, but also of bacteria that are resistant to many different antibiotics. As the resistances accumulate, they can be found on one or two plasmids in the bacterial cell. These can be transferred all together to other bacteria. So one new recipient cell can receive the entire resistance "package" of another bacterium. The net result is that many previously powerful, nontoxic, inexpensive, and often lifesaving antibiotics can become useless quickly.

*   *   *   *   *

Individual users and physicians frequently abuse antibiotics, but neither is the only culprit. In many instances, it is others making decisions for the individual whom we should fault for their ignorance of the ramifications of such abuse. Under a rationale of prophylaxis, that is, preventive treatment, many well-meaning people are providing antibiotics to tens of thousands of people. Whether it is the mother from a Boston suburb who innocently treats a busload of children with penicillin because one of them has a cold, or a government agency in Indonesia that authorizes giving tetracycline to thousands going on a pilgrimage, the result is the same—killing of sensitive bacteria and recruitment of resistant types.

"One hundred thousand people, pilgrims, are going to Mecca this month," the laboratory technician told me while I was visiting Jakarta, Indonesia. He was referring to a hundred thousand people from all parts of Indonesia who would be traveling by foot, train, and plane. The pilgrimage, a massive trek to Saudi Arabia, was, to many of these people, their lifelong dream, and they were determined to make it. The rich and the poor went together. Only their mode of transportation distinguished one from the other.

However, the Indonesian Ministry of Religion, which organized and directed the pilgrimage, was concerned about the possible spread of disease among these people. The most likely devastating disease was cholera. This severe form of diarrhea, caused by the bacterium *Vibrio cholerae*, often spreads among people via contaminated water or food or through close physical contact. For this reason, all foods served on the trains and planes were checked for these disease-causing bacteria, as well as for *Salmonella*, another potential cause of diarrhea. The laboratory I was visiting in 1981 was responsible for these analyses.

Many lives had been lost to infectious diseases during these pilgrimages. So a new approach had been developed whereby each individual was checked for cholera before departure. And then, just in case, each was given the antibiotic tetracycline.

"You mean all 100,000 pilgrims are getting tetracycline?" I asked in a state of disbelief.

"Yes, and for seven days," replied my host. "In fact, the government keeps them in quarantine for this period until they finish taking the drug."

He told me that the Ministry of Religion supplies the antibiotic. It is "dished out of vats like coffee beans." I already knew the answer to my next question but asked anyway. "Is there any control on the quality of the drug?" When antibiotics are given in bulk, it is often necessary to confirm that the drug is fully active. He told me that this was the job of the Food and Drug Administration, but that agency was not involved in the pilgrimage.

This broad-scale use of tetracycline, to "prevent" illness by trying to kill off any infectious bacteria that *might* be there, misses certain key features in the infectious process. First, one microorganism does not cause disease; there must be thousands to millions of them. Second, antibiotics will provide a selective environment for those infectious agents that are resistant to them. Those bacteria that happen to enter our bodies or fall onto our skin take up residence and multiply to dangerously high numbers, all under antibiotic protection. Widespread use of tetracycline has certainly contributed to the increasing number of tetracycline-resistant strains of *V. cholerae* that plague large areas of the developing world. In certain areas, such as parts of Africa, over 50% of the cholera-causing bacteria are now resistant to tetracycline. This antibiotic has always been the drug of choice for treating this disease. Substitute drugs are being tried, but many strains are now becoming resistant to these as well.

Prior to the 1970s, the cholera bacteria were uniformly susceptible to all these drugs. The resistance they have gained had its origins in other kinds of bacteria, such as *E. coli*, which normally live in the gut. By some transfer event, resistances have moved from their previous hosts to new ones, namely to the *Vibrio cholerae* bacterium.

*   *   *   *   *

In the United States, the ease with which an individual can procure antibiotics from physicians and then stockpile them for self-prescription later on, is a variation on the same theme we see happening in developing countries. And the numbers of individuals abusing antibiotics here in the United States can be counted in the hundreds of thousands.

Dr. T., an energetic and outgoing psychologist, was tired at the end of her work day, especially after the last, tedious, hour-long session with one of her many clients. She took off to a popular bar near her office in Boston. At age 31 and unmarried, she enjoyed chance meetings during these "after hours" relaxations. On this evening, Mr. S., carrying a draft beer, made his way through the crowd and stopped next to her. "Hi, may I join you?" he asked. Dr. T. was delighted. He looked about her age, maybe a little younger. Their drink together was followed by dinner and then a nightcap at her place. It was not surprising to either of them that they found themselves in bed. Dr. T. was not reluctant, but the fear of unexpected infection could have been a deterrent if it hadn't been for her supply of ampicillin tablets, her choice of antibiotic protection. She had diligently kept a supply on hand from previous prescriptions for those evenings spent with someone different. She took two pills before and two after. "You never know with whom you might be sleeping!"

This story predates the problem of AIDS but provides a glimpse of an attitude about antibiotic misuse that persists. It's the self-treatment syndrome combined with the ready availability of antibiotics for self-medication by the individual. Even in the United States this occurs, although there are laws requiring prescriptions to procure these drugs. As far as we know, Dr. T. continues today to use antibiotics on her own, despite our advice to the contrary.

Appropriate use of antibiotics is straightforward and involves the prescription of the drug by a physician to kill off bacteria invading the body of the patient. Clear directives for the use of these drugs come together with the prescription and should be well within the awareness of these educated self-prescribers. But apparently, directives don't provide enough incentive to prompt proper use of antibiotics. Abuse is rampant. This pattern of abuse contributes to the alarming frequency with which resistant bacteria are appearing as causes of disease.

Antibiotics have two major acceptable uses in medicine— treatment and prophylaxis (Figure 5.2). In the area of treatment, antibiotics are given when a known infectious microorganism causes disease. Here the choice can be geared to the microorganism and its expected susceptibility. Another, and perhaps the most common use, is when a bacterial infection is highly suspected by the physician, even though the microorganism has not yet been identified. In this instance, an antibiotic is chosen based on the best clinical judgment. Obviously, it is in this area where there is more room for misuse. Antibiotics are also recommended for disease prophylaxis, that is, to prevent infection at times when there is a known high risk of contracting an infectious illness. Unfortunately, in reality, neither users nor prescribers confine their involvement with antibiotics to only these two conditions.

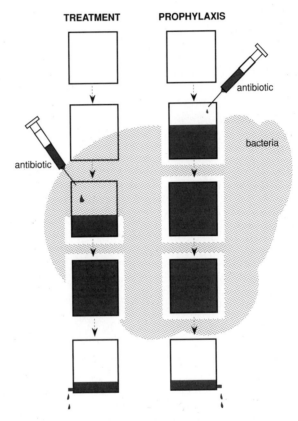

Figure 5.2. Antibiotics have two major roles in the control of infectious diseases: treatment and prophylaxis. The major difference is the timing of the antibiotic. In treatment, the antibiotic is applied after the infection is already present. In prophylaxis, the antibiotic is applied first, preventing infection by invading bacteria such as during certain surgical procedures (Bonnie Marshall, Tufts University School of Medicine).

SELECTING AN ANTIBIOTIC

In the early days of antibiotic discovery, drugs such as penicillin, tetracycline, and streptomycin were developed because of their recognized and unique efficacy against particular disease-causing microorganisms. As more of these antibiotics became available, they were tried on other diseases. Thus the spectrum of bacteria that they killed was established and, in many cases, broadened.

Today we speak of "broad" and "narrow" spectrum antibiotics in reference to the long or short list of bacterial types affected by the drug. Penicillin, which originally provided a narrow use, has been chemically altered to produce other derivatives that are more broadly effective. Pharmaceutical companies were able to take penicillin's chemical core structure and modify it, thus enlarging its spectrum of activity. Certain penicillin modifications improved the drug's ability to penetrate the outer cell wall of other previously untouchable bacteria. These bacteria included the dreaded *Pseudomonas aeruginosa*, which plagues patients with blood diseases and those undergoing cancer therapy. Practitioners valued the new derivatives for their extended use in killing off yet other kinds of bacteria.

Chemists also modified the core penicillin molecule in order to produce a new kind of penicillin that was not subject to certain resistance mechanisms. The product, methicillin, was not destroyed by enzymes that degraded penicillin in resistant cells. This altered penicillin was able to kill the resistant staphylococcus bacteria which made the penicillin-destroying enzymes.

Today, we have over a hundred antibiotics from which to choose (Table 5.1). Interestingly, penicillin and tetracycline, the first antibiotics to be discovered, are still in great use today. This practice reflects, in part, the success of chemical modifications that broaden their activities and counteract resistance. To some extent, this continued use stems from the dilemma of poorer countries where the newer drugs are too expensive to be widely used.

Table 5.1. Representative antibiotics and antibacterials used in human therapy.[a]

Penicillins	Cephalosporins	β-lactam inhibitors (used in combination with penicillins)
V, VK	1st-generation	Clavulanic acid
Phenoxymethylpenicillin	Cephalothin	Sulbactam
Phenoxymethylpenicillin potassium	Cephalexin	**Thienamycin**
G	Cephradine	Imipenem
Benzylpenicillin	Cefaclor	**Monobactams**
Benethamine penicillin	Cefadroxil	Aztreonam
Procaine penicillin	Cephapirin	**Chloramphenicol**
Broad-spectrum	2nd-generation	**Tetracyclines**
Ampicillin	Cefazolin	Tetracycline
Amoxicillin	Cefoxitin	Demeclocycline
Bacampicillin	Cefuroxime	Doxycycline
Carbenicillin	Cefamandole	Methacycline
Ticarcillin	Cefmetazole	Minocycline
Azlocillin	3rd-generation	Oxytetracycline
Mezlocillin	Cefoperazone	Chlortetracycline
Piperacillin	Cefotaxime	
Antistaphylococcal	Cefsulodin	
Nafcillin	Cefotetan	
Methicillin	Ceftazidime	
Oxacillin	Ceftriaxone	
Dicloxacillin	Cefixime	
	Ceftizoxime	

Aminoglycosides
Streptomycin
Kanamycin
Paromomycin
Neomycin
Gentamicin
Tobramycin
Netilmicin
Amikacin
Macrolides
Erythromycin
Azithromycin
Clarithromycin
Lincosamides
Lincomycin
Clindamycin

Quinolones
Nalidixic acid
Oxolinic acid
Ciprofloxacin
Norfloxacin
Pefloxacin
Ofloxacin
Sulfonamides
Sulfacytine
Sulfadiazine
Sulfamethizole
Sulfamethoxazole
Sulfapyridine
Sulfasalazine
Sulfisoxazole
Trisulfapyrimidines
Trimethoprim

Antituberculosis agents
p-Aminosalicylic acid
Capreomycin
Cycloserine
Ethambutol
Ethionamide
Isoniazid
Pyrazinamide
Rifampin
Urinary antibacterial agents
Nitrofurantoin
Methenamine
Other Antibiotics
Vancomycin
Bacitracin
Colistin
Polymyxin B
Spectinomycin
Novobiocin
Metronidazole
Fosfomycin

[a]Adapted from Col and O'Connor 1987.

Often, the first-line drugs are all that are available, despite their known failure rates against resistant bacteria.

The challenge for the physician is to know when and for what kind of bacteria a particular antibiotic should be prescribed. Fever usually indicates invasion of the body by a foreign agent, be it bacterium or virus. It is unusual, unless the individual's body defenses are subdued by anti-inflammatory drugs that mask fever, for a bacterial infection in the blood, lungs, or other major site in the body, not to cause fever. Therefore, without fever, antibiotics, as systemic drugs, should be prescribed sparingly. There are, of course, exceptions. Local infections, such as skin abscesses or impetigo, which is a more superficial skin infection, are usually caused by bacteria and should be treated with antibiotics, even though no fever may be present. Sinusitis, especially in children, which lasts more than ten days, has a good chance of being bacterial since viral outbreaks usually improve within a week. Fever may not be present. In this instance, antibiotics are recommended because of the high probability of a bacterial cause.

If a bacterial infection is suspected, further diagnostic procedures are generally implemented. A physician will want to identify the specific microorganism before purging the body with large doses of antibiotic. Knowing the kind of bacteria causing the disease helps the physician decide what kind of disease symptoms and signs to expect and what kind of drug to use. Certain bacteria have propensities to infect certain organs, such as the heart, lung, or kidney. Some antibiotics are more effective when given for a bacterial infection of a particular organ because the antibiotic is concentrated in the fluid of that organ, such as the urine in the kidney or the bile in the gallbladder.

To secure this information, physicians obtain cultures and perform tests of different areas of the body. In the presence of fever and soreness of the throat or difficulty in swallowing, a physician may want to obtain a swab of the throat and culture it to check for a bacterial culprit, such as streptococcus, which causes "strep throat" or scarlet fever (Figure 5.3). If the person has a deep cough, suggestive of a lung infection, one or more samples of the cough

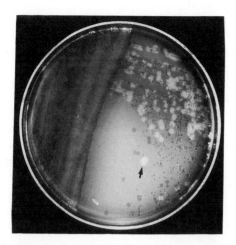

Figure 5.3. The agar plate is an important tool in the work-up of an infectious disease. In this instance, a throat culture is swabbed onto a blood agar plate and the colonies are separated to be visualized and identified. The β-hemolytic strep-tococcus, which causes "strep throat," produces a protein that lyses the animal blood cells suspended in the agar. This is visualized as a halo around the streptococcus colony (arrow).

secretions, or sputum, are taken and tested for the presence of a known disease-causing bacterium. Initially, a simple test can be done in the office. The sputum sample is smeared on a glass slide that is stained for bacteria, namely by the Gram stain. The pres-ence of small, round, purple-stained bacteria in chains of two cells, called diplococci, are highly suggestive of pneumococci, which cause so-called "lobar" pneumonia in one or more parts of the lung. With this evidence, and an X-ray confirming pneu-monia, the physician would initiate treatment, either at home or in the hospital, depending on the severity of the pneumonia. Defini-tive identity of the microorganism and an antibiotic susceptibility test would come from culturing the sputum.

If there is burning on urination or pain in the flank areas where the kidneys are located, the physician can usually detect a kidney or bladder infection by direct microscopic viewing of a urine sediment obtained by centrifuging a sample of freshly voided urine. Urine cultures are important in confirming the diagnosis and determining the kind of microorganism involved, including its susceptibility to antibiotics.

Loose or watery bowel movements and cramps lasting a week or more or bloody diarrhea would suggest the need of a stool specimen. These tests tell us about dysenterylike microorganisms, such as *Shigella* or *Campylobacter*, or microorganisms causing milder diarrhea, such as *Vibrio cholerae* and *Salmonella*. Perhaps it is not a bacterial cause at all, but rather a parasite, such as *Giardia*.

A careful examination of the skin, including the perianal area, will often tell the observer whether or not there is a deep-seated skin infection that needs to be cultured in order to help decide on a treatment regimen.

If no particular organ or area of the body seems to be the problem and the patient is feverish and appears generally ill, three separate cultures of blood are performed. Since a blood-borne infection would need immediate attention, such patients would usually be transferred to the hospital for these tests and for further evaluation and treatment. The need to check multiple blood samples has come from studies showing that bacteria, even when present, may not be discovered in a given culture all the time.

All clinical specimens go to a bacteriology laboratory where they are put into culture systems that allow growth of any microorganisms present. In the case of blood, bacteriologists inoculate some of the specimen into bottles of growth media, a mixture of salts and nutrients, in order to allow the small numbers of bacteria present to reach detectable levels. Since all internal body samples should be sterile, any growth in the bottles containing blood samples indicates a blood-borne infection. Cultures of urine, feces, and skin all contain normal bacterial inhabitants that must be distinguished from any that could be the cause of the disease. This distinction is made by inoculating the specimens onto a special gelatin medium (like the agar plate first described by Koch in the last century) in round plastic dishes. This plating promotes easy growth of the bacteria into separate colonies and allows identification of the numbers and types of bacteria present in the specimen. In samples from nonsterile sites, the bacteriologist or medical technologist looks discerningly to recognize the harmful bacteria mixed among bacteria normally present in this body material. Certain special tests may be needed to aid in this distinction. For some infections of the bowel or abdomen, bacteria that die in air, the so-called strict anaerobes, may be causing the infection. Therefore, some of the cultures are grown in the presence of nitrogen rather than oxygen.

If the bacteriology laboratory finds disease-causing bacteria in these samples, the microorganism is usually tested for its susceptibility to antibiotics. Before our present-day problem with antibiotic resistance, simple identification of the type of bacteria causing the disease would have been enough to tell the physician which antibiotic to use. Nowadays we must also determine which antibiotic is likely to be successful.

In many United States hospitals, susceptibility testing is done by an automated machine. Bacteriologists inoculate small amounts of bacteria growing in a medium into separate tubes of a liquid test growth solution, each containing a different antibiotic. If growth occurs in the tube containing an antibiotic, the bacteria are resistant to that antibiotic. Alternatively, some laboratories test by using paper discs (Figure 5.4). The bacteriologist swabs a solution of suspect bacteria onto the surface of an agar plate and lays small paper discs containing antibiotics on top. After a day of incubation at 37°C (98°F), the temperature of the human body, the technologist examines the plates and measures the area around the antibiotic disc where bacteria have not grown. If there is a large area with no lawn of bacteria, the strain is designated susceptible to the antibiotic in that disc. If there is growth close to the edge of the disc, the strain is resistant. The bacteriology laboratory reports these results to the clinician seeing the patient (Figure 5.5). On the basis of these susceptibility tests, the physician makes his choice of antibiotic.

The physician must always make a choice of antibiotic based

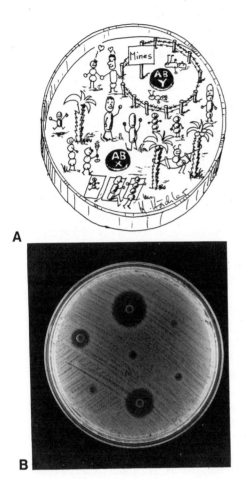

Figure 5.4. Antibiotic testing is done in several different ways; the most widely used is the paper disc method. Paper discs impregnated with the antibiotic are placed onto an agar medium already spread with a lawn of the bacteria being tested. During overnight incubation, the antibiotic diffuses into the agar, killing susceptible bacteria. Clear zones around the paper disc indicate bacterial sensitivity to the antibiotic. Growth up to the edge of the disc indicates resistance to the antibiotic. In the cartoon (plate A) the bacteria are resistant to AB-X but susceptible to AB-Y. Plate B contains *E. coli* from an Indonesian infant with diarrhea. On this plate, the bacteria are susceptible to gentamicin and sulfamethoxazole, moderately susceptible to kanamycin, but resistant to ampicillin, tetracycline, chloramphenicol, and streptomycin. (Cartoon by Herbert Hächler, University of Zurich, Zurich, Switzerland.)

not only on the susceptibility results, but also from knowledge of possible allergies of the patient. There is also consideration for the method by which the drug has to be given (orally or parenterally, i.e. by injection into the vein or muscle). Increasingly, although not frequently enough, physicians will also look at the costs of the

```
 07/05/90 D 1915        3235
CULTURE WOUND
SOURCE                  RIGHT FOOT
DATE FINAL REPORT       7/08
PRELIM. ORGANISM 1      MANY STAPHYLOCOCCUS SPECIES
FINAL   ORGANISM 1      MANY STAPHYLOCOCCUS AUREUS
PRELIM. ORGANISM 2
FINAL   ORGANISM 2      MODERATE DIPHTHEROIDS

ORGANISM NUMBER                 1
AMPICILLIN/SULBACTAM               >=32 R
CEPHALOTHIN                        >=32 R
CIPROFLOXACIN                       >=4 R
CLINDAMYCIN                         >=8 R
ERYTHROMYCIN                        >=8 R
OXACILLIN                          >=8 R
PENICILLIN                         >=16 R
TRIMETH/SULFA                      <=10 S
VANCOMYCIN                           1 S
MIC VALUE IN MCG/ML
```

Figure 5.5. An antibiotic susceptibility report on a patient with a bone infection. *Staphylococcus aureus* was isolated and showed multidrug resistance, including resistance to one of the newer quinolones, ciprofloxacin. The microorganism was still susceptible to the combination of trimethoprim and sulfamethoxazole and to vancomycin, which, in this case, was the drug of choice.

drugs tested. If two drugs are equally effective, the physician will choose the less expensive. Cost has only recently become a major consideration, in large part because of the high price of some of the newer drugs. For instance, a penicillin treatment typically costs less than a dollar a day, whereas some of the newer antibiotics could cost over one hundred dollars.

In general, use of a single antibiotic is the optimal choice. This avoids problems with side effects, since any one drug can have a side effect and many different side effects could follow use of multiple drugs. Some side effects are expected and occur in most consumers of the antibiotic—these are usually mild and can be tolerated. Others are less common and indicate an allergic reaction—these could be serious. In our population, allergy to drugs is relatively common, second only to hay fever allergy. About 5% of the population may show a reaction to penicillin. While most often this is only a rash, sometimes the reaction can be more severe and the rash may be a warning sign. The antibiotic should be stopped immediately.

The situation can become even more difficult when some penicillin-allergic people show reactions to other drugs with structures related to penicillin. Thus, the physician has to be careful in selecting the alternative drugs. If a patient is taking more than one antibiotic and a rash or other adverse reaction develops, it is impossible to know which antibiotic is the cause. Consequently, all drugs must be stopped and a new one needs to be started. When several antibiotics are suspected of being the cause of the reaction, the search for an alternative effective drug will be more difficult.

The decision to use an antibiotic is based generally, in the best medical hands, on the benefits compared with the risks associated with its use. In a sick infant suffering from fever and possible dehydration and having little body resilience, the high probability of bacterial infection warrants the use of antibiotics immediately and for the sustained period of the illness. In this case, early use of these drugs can be truly lifesaving. Still, clinicians will take cultures of affected areas—throat, urine, feces—before starting the antibiotic to confirm that the right drug has been started. Sometimes, the initial antibiotic taken may not cure the disease and another will have to be given. However, the microorganisms may have been suppressed in this process. If cultures were not taken prior to starting the first antibiotic, it may be too late at this point to culture and identify the bacteria causing the disease. Thus, there will be no susceptibility test from which to choose an appropriate alternative drug.

In severely ill infants, we are willing to accept possible side effects and biological changes in bacterial flora resulting from antibiotic use because the benefit far exceeds the risk. By a similar reasoning, an elderly, very sick patient with high fever and other signs of obvious infection is presumed to have a bacterial infection. Therefore, after culturing possible sites of infection, antibiotics are begun. The risk of rampant disease in this setting is too great to wait for the culture results. The same decision is not appropriate, however, for an otherwise healthy, young adult who suffers from symptoms attributable to a suspected viral illness. Here, there is time for culturing and waiting the necessary 24 hours for the culture results before beginning an antibiotic. This reasoning is not meant to deny appropriate therapy. It should prevent unnecessary side effects for the individual and remove a purposeless selection of resistant strains for the community, not to mention saving costs for an already overburdened health care system.

ANTIBIOTICS IN DISEASE PREVENTION

Aside from their use in treating disease, antibiotics have a proper place in preventing threatening bacterial disease. About 30–50% of all antibiotics dispensed in the United States are used for this purpose. The use of penicillin for the victims of the Cocoanut Grove fire in the 1940s was a mixture of therapy and prophylaxis. Some received the drug for infection already present; others were given the antibiotic to prevent infection during skin grafting.

A common prophylactic use of antibiotics is to prevent infection in patients who have had diseases of the valves of their heart or have a heart murmur. The latter indicates some change in the normal functioning of the heart valves that may make them more susceptible to bacterial infections. Damaged valves are at increased risk of infections whenever bacteria circulate in the blood. This can occur, for instance, following tooth extractions that might cause transient passage of bacteria from the mouth into the bloodstream. Antibiotics cannot prevent the bacteria from entering the bloodstream, but they can prevent them from "setting up shop." This preventive effect of antibiotics does not need to be prolonged.

Therefore, this use is for short periods of time before and immediately after a dental procedure.

Some serious diseases in small children, such as meningitis caused by an invasive type of *Hemophilus* or the meningococcus often suggest the need for prophylactic use of antibiotics in schoolmates as well as household contacts. This practice is done to halt the spread of these life-threatening infections.

Antibiotics are sometimes used to prevent recurrent infections, namely lobar pneumonia caused by pneumococci, in people who have had their spleens removed for therapy or for rupture after trauma. The spleen produces antibodies that are protective against the bacteria that cause these pneumonias. When the spleen is gone, an antibiotic is often advocated. Today, this practice is being replaced by vaccination against different types of pneumococci and other bacteria before removal of the spleen. Similarly, children who have had rheumatic fever caused by a streptococcus may be maintained for years on penicillin. This practice has been shown to prevent recurrent streptococcus infection, and in particular, to protect against serious damage to the heart.

Medical practitioners and surgeons know that antibiotics can be extremely useful in preventing postsurgical infections. These are limited to operations which involve locations and tissues that have a high risk of bacterial contamination, such as operations on the intestinal tract or following trauma with external contaminated objects. For this use, the effectiveness of the antibiotic as a prophylactic agent is, almost by definition, limited to the short period of time before, during, and sometimes immediately after surgery. A physician need not prescribe any additional drugs beyond this protective period since the chance of infection from the surgical procedure is over. It is important not to continue these drugs beyond this period unless there is clear evidence of infection. Prolonged use can select for infectious agents circulating in hospitals that are often resistant and emerge in the presence of the antibiotic. Besides the medical consequences to the patient, unnecessary antibiotic use is a major contributor to increased hospitalization costs.

Prophylactic use of antibiotics is less rigid in practice since it is based on suspected risk rather than known disease. Therefore, there is room for more error and, in some cases, blatant misuse. In a study of surgery patients in over 50 hospitals in Pennsylvania during the late 1970s, investigators found that, for a large proportion of patients, prophylactic use of antibiotics for surgery was not limited to the short period before and during surgery but instead was prolonged for the entire hospital stay. This amounted to weeks of antibiotic misuse and long periods of potential selection of antibiotic resistant strains in these individuals and in the hospital. In cases such as this one, where there was no need for the antibiotic, such continued use tends to lead to the killing off of susceptible harmless bacteria that normally protect us from invasion by other harmful varieties of bacteria. The scenario can be likened to feeding your lawn with weed killer, only to find that the grass is killed off as well; the small number of weeds that survive or enter right after the treatment now have a wide-open area to seed and spread, unimpeded by natural competitors (Figure 5.6).

Fortunately, documentation of this source of misuse and recognition of its harm both biologically and economically has led to vast changes in surgical prophylaxis. Antibiotic prophylaxis is generally not recommended for "clean" operations except where the rare chance of infection could produce drastic consequences, such as in heart surgery. For contaminated or potentially contaminated procedures, prophylaxis is indicated. Data have fully substantiated the success of the prophylaxis. In a recent study, the timing of antibiotic prophylaxis was found to be crucial—two hours or less before the incision produced the best results. When the antibiotic was given more than two hours before or after the incision, the benefit was less. If the procedure is expected to last for more than four hours, a second dose is recommended, generally within two hours of the first dose. While some believe that no further prophylaxis is required after termination of the operative

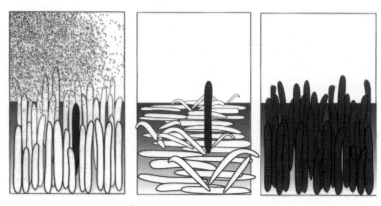

Figure 5.6. Antibiotics kill more than the pathogen to which they are directed. The growth of any other susceptible bacteria will also be inhibited. Once the ecosystem is cleared of bacteria, resistant bacteria can multiply or enter into the noncompetitive arena. The phenomenon can be likened to weeds that have overgrown a lawn where the grass has been completely destroyed by an overdose of herbicides (Bonnie Marshall, Tufts University School of Medicine).

procedure, others accept a limit of no more than 24 hours following the end of the procedure.

RESISTANCE IN THE COMMUNITY: A CONSEQUENCE OF ANTIBIOTIC USE AND AVAILABILITY

Urinary tract infections are common, particularly in women. An estimated 40% of the female population will have the problem at least once in their lifetimes. The infecting bacteria usually come from the gut where they find entry into the bladder through the neighboring urethra. As we discussed earlier, when antibiotics are taken, the susceptible strains of bacteria on human skin, mucous membranes, nasal passages and in the gastrointestinal tract are killed off by the onslaught of an antibiotic (and in many cases by more than one), leaving room for chance colonization by harmful strains. The longer the use, the greater the effect on our natural flora. Thus, the antibiotic susceptibility of the bowel flora could affect the treatment of a urinary tract infection. Not all bacteria can cause urinary tract infections. To some extent it is the chance meeting of one type of bacterium with the vulnerable anatomy of a "susceptible" person. There are, for example, some women who will not get an infection even if the potential disease-causing agent is there. In other less usual instances, the infection occurs. The so-called "honeymoon cystitis" is attributed to spread of fecal bacteria to the bladder during periods of frequent sexual activity.

While infections of the bladder are usually easily and successfully treated with antibiotics, some can present real difficulties if the infecting microorganism is resistant. A young woman from Kenya who had had ready access there to all currently available antibiotics came to Boston for consultation because she had a persistent urinary tract infection that did not respond to antibiotics. Once again, the culprit infectious agent was a multiply-resistant common gut bacterium. Only when treated by intravenous therapy with expensive and somewhat toxic drugs, to which she had never been exposed, was she cured of her infection. Time alone will show us for how long.

In some patients, one potential way for treating persistent urinary tract infection is to rid the intestinal tract of the causative bacteria so that the patient will not become reinfected with the same strain. But this poses strategic problems—we cannot sterilize the gut. However, a change of diet might work, since changes in diet, along with bacteria associated normally with the food, can affect the kinds of bacteria that reside in our intestinal tract. In fact, some bacterial strains in our intestinal tract are constantly in flux. If one of these strains is the cause of the urinary tract infection, we can try to get rid of it. To this end, some people suggest eating yogurt. Its efficacy comes from its containing lactobacillus, a common intestinal microorganism that causes us no harm but colonizes the intestinal tract and, in doing so, can change the flora. Lactobacillus has been advocated and used to help reestablish the normal intestinal flora after antibiotic treatment. We now know that it is not necessarily any one type of lactobacillus that can help produce this change. Intestinal microbiologists and physicians are presently working on particular strains of lactobacillus that appear to be more effective than others. It may be, as certain animal studies suggest, that lactobacillus can even help rid the intestine of *E. coli* causing diarrhea and perhaps other human ailments, such as bladder infection. We can expect to hear more about these strains in the future.

A female employee of a Boston hospital had such a persistent urinary tract infection that she was almost constantly on some form of antibiotic treatment. While a cure was usually attained eventually, each treatment required a different antibiotic. Whenever the drugs were stopped, however, the infection resurged. The infection recurred with either the same microorganism or with one showing a new resistance pattern. We advised her to change the place where she normally ate, a local cafeteria, on the chance that her intestinal flora would change, leading to the loss of those microorganisms causing her repeated bladder infections. By coincidence, or by the direct effect of her changing eating establishments, her bladder infections ceased when she stopped eating lunch at this cafeteria. Whether the problem was the bacteria associated with the food she was ingesting or her own intestinal flora that this previous diet encouraged is not clear, but the change in diet appeared to place the bacteria causing her disease at a disadvantage—at least they did not return to bother her. Our interpretation was that she finally eliminated the infecting resistant strains that were constantly recolonizing her gut and causing her urinary tract infections.

A common example of a community-acquired resistant bacterial infection that has emerged under antibiotic selection is the gonococcus bacterium that causes the venereal disease gonorrhea. Previously, penicillin offered an easy cure, but the bacteria have now become resistant to this first-line antibiotic. As noted earlier, this emergence of resistance in a widespread infectious agent in the mid 1970s caused eyebrows to raise and previous doubters to take heed. Antibiotic resistance was not just limited to a few hospital strains or normal intestinal inhabitants. The initial appearance of resistance to penicillin in this microorganism was so new that it allowed the resistant forms to be traced to the brothels of Southeast Asia, one of the aftermaths of the Vietnam war. It was a common practice there for penicillin to be given to women on a regular basis to prevent venereal disease, thereby protecting their servicemen customers. While not proven, the likelihood is that the first resistant gonococcus appeared in Vietnam and was soon transported to Singapore, Europe, and the rest of the world. Today, every country in the world has to deal with this new resistant form of a bacterium which was previously susceptible to penicillin.

The rise in penicillin resistance in the gonococcus microorganism necessitated a change to tetracycline, always the second-line agent for patients allergic to penicillin. But today tetracycline is also becoming less and less useful in the face of increasing numbers of tetracycline-resistant gonococcal strains. Their appearance was first documented in New Hampshire in the United States in 1982, but they were discovered soon in other eastern states. Epidemiologists see them spreading worldwide. Isolates have already emerged in the Netherlands and other parts of Europe. A sizeable number of these recently resistant gonococci are multiresistant, that is, resistant to both tetracycline and penicillin. This situation has caused New York State public health officials and the Centers for Disease Control to recommend using yet another antibiotic, a newer type of cephalosporin, as the drug of choice in treating suspected gonorrhea. This is unfortunate since this drug, in contrast to tetracycline, will not simultaneously treat other venereal disease agents that might also be involved. The antibiotic is also more than three times as expensive as tetracycline or penicillin.

Another now common community resistance problem has developed with *Hemophilus influenzae*, the cause of ear infections in infants, as well as of pneumonia, and of meningitis, the infection of the tissue covering the brain. The first appearance of ampicillin-resistant strains was totally unexpected. They were discovered in the early 1970s when two infants in Bethesda, Maryland failed to respond to ampicillin. They both died before the problem of resistance was diagnosed. The event sparked international concern. But these strains had already begun to appear elsewhere. At the time, Londoners were cautioned about picking up the bacteria from Americans stationed there. In a letter to *Nature* about the potential spread of this resistant *Hemophilus*, the authors warned,

> Since there is considerable intermingling of the American military community with our British hosts, the above data [increased numbers of ampicillin-resistant *Hemophilus* in the UK] suggest the distinct possibility that the American community may act as a source of ampicillin-resistant invasive *H. influenzae* disease for the community at large.[1]

Today, less than twenty years later, ampicillin-resistant and multiresistant *Hemophilus influenzae* is a problem throughout the world.

A more recent example of troubling susceptibility changes involves the Group A β-hemolytic streptococcus. This microorganism causes strep throat, scarlet fever, rheumatic fever, and many other illnesses in children and adults. It was, in fact, the microorganism *Streptococcus pyogenes* that took the life of Jim Henson, the creator of the popular Muppets© of "Sesame Street" fame. Fortunately for us, all group A streptococci are still susceptible to penicillin, the drug of first choice, and treatment is successful when begun soon after infection. However, there has been an alarming increase in resistance of this microorganism to the second drug of choice for treatment—erythromycin.

Erythromycin-resistant group A streptococci were reported more than a decade ago in Japan and other reports have come out of Canada and Australia. However, they have never reached levels of sustained clinical concern. In Japan, the frequency went down when erythromycin usage was reduced. An important study recently conducted in Finland discovered a dramatic increase in erythromycin-resistant *S. pyogenes* in 1990. The study was initiated two years before, when many erythromycin-resistant isolates from throat swabs were noted in Turku, on the southwestern coast of Finland. The authors established a prospective study to examine whether this was a one-time event or an increasing phenomenon in Finland. The latter concern turned out to be disturbingly true— the problem did not go away and, in fact, was escalating. They made some important observations. There had been more than a threefold increase in the sale of erythromycin in Finland over the previous decade. They also showed that erythromycin-resistant bacteria were the cause of disease in half the patients who did not respond to erythromycin treatment, a finding vastly different from the 96% of patients cured of the disease who carried a susceptible strain.

There are several important points that follow from these data. First, a microorganism that causes a common illness worldwide has moved from being highly susceptible to one that is able to resist at least one of the key drugs important in its treatment. For those who are allergic to penicillin, erythromycin is the drug of second choice. Erythromycin is also helpful in the treatment of other disease agents that could complicate upper respiratory tract disease. Secondly, we see that resistance frequency increased rapidly in this location over the three-year period from 1988 to 1990 and has been sustained since then. The authors suggest that limiting erythromycin use, as was done in Japan, might help bring the resistance levels down. However, as we noted before, once a resistant strain, such as an erythromycin-resistant *Streptococcus pyogenes*, emerges in high frequency, it may find its niche alongside the susceptible strains and stay. From there, it can reemerge under erythromycin selection. There is also the potential of this resistant microorganism spreading to other parts of the world. Finally, as a consequence of this emergence, more routine antibiotic susceptibility testing is required, particularly if a person is allergic to penicillinlike drugs.

The early recognition of resistance to penicillin in the 1940s heralded a phenomenon now seen commonly with the introduction of each new antibiotic. We practice medicine differently now than in the past. More emphasis than ever is placed on rapid diagnosis and susceptibility testing of the infectious microorganism. While antibiotics are needed and provide immeasurable power to control infectious diseases, their widespread use, often in inappropriate ways and amounts, has contributed to the emergence and rise of resistant bacteria. Given the strong selection of resistant variants by these drugs, the judicious use of antibiotics must become an even greater priority for both the prescriber and the consumer.

Chapter 6

ANTIBIOTICS, ANIMALS, AND THE RESISTANCE GENE POOL

Of the six billion animals raised for human consumption in the United States yearly, most receive some antibiotics during their short lifetimes. In any one year, domestic food animals outnumber humans in the United States by more than five to one. These figures are important when we assess the effect that antibiotics have on the bacterial flora of these animals that not only share our environment, but also end up in our stomachs.

Just as is the case with people, antibiotics are given to domesticated animals for treatment of disease. But quantitatively, much greater amounts of antibiotics are given to animals in small, subtherapeutic levels as a means to improve their growth. When considered in terms of nationwide use, the amount of this subtherapeutic usage is four to five times greater than the amount used for treatment of animal diseases. Antibiotics are also used to treat illnesses in domestic pets, such as dogs and cats, adding another 100–150 million animals to the total number ingesting antibiotics.

In the years following the early success of antibiotics in curing human infections, veterinarians—as well as food producers—looked to these drugs as the answer to infectious disease problems facing livestock. They were not disappointed. The results were so dramatic that antibiotics were soon credited for curing diseases of all kinds, including viral illnesses. This latter claim persists today, even though we now know that antibiotics do not cure viral infections. Most likely, these early observers had treated infections caused by bacteria, not viruses.

In the early 1950s, doses below therapeutic amounts began to be introduced into animal feeds for growth enhancement at about the same time that antibiotics were introduced therapeutically for animals. The discovery of the beneficial effects of small amounts of antibiotics came during the period when food animal producers were searching for "nutritional factors," such as new vitamins, that would improve the growth rate of their animals. Nor was this search limited to animals. There was even a quest to identify factors that would improve the growth of children, particularly in poorer areas of the world where food supplies were limited. A serendipitous discovery propelled the subtherapeutic use of antibiotics as growth promoters into the animal husbandry field.

Robert Stokstad, Thomas Jukes, and colleagues were looking for new microbial sources of "animal protein factor," later found to be vitamin B_{12}, that would improve efficacy of protein utilization and growth in chickens. They were working at Lederle Laboratories, where, in 1947, Benjamin Duggar discovered chlortetracycline, the first member of the tetracycline family of antibiotics. Procuring this drug required harvesting large vats of *Streptomyces aureofaciens*, the soil microorganisms producing the antibiotic. When these investigators tested the microorganism itself, they discovered that it contained a growth enhancer, at first thought to be vitamin B_{12}. But the response was greater than any seen with other vitamin B_{12} sources. Moreover, when chlortetracycline had been extracted from the microorganisms and the leftover carcasses of the tiny bacterial cells were given to the animals, the growth effect was retained. This meant that the growth promoting agent was not lost during extraction of the antibiotic. These investigators realized that this material represented an inexpensive source of the "animal protein factor" as well as a growth enhancer for chickens and other animals. Their studies showed that adding even small amounts of the *Streptomyces* mash to chicken feed led to a significant increase in the growth rate of the chickens and weight gain per pound of feed. They initially attributed this effect to a new nutritional "growth factor." They later found that it was nothing other than traces of chlortetracycline remaining in the bacterial carcasses after extraction—in an amount of about 1–5 parts per million. The potential of such small amounts of antibiotic to improve growth was a powerful discovery that generated a whole new industry. Because of the extremely small amounts of antibiotic, this effect of chlortetracycline was regarded as "nutritional" and not therapeutic by the producers and governmental authorities regulating the food industry. This seemingly innocent interpretation allowed these antibiotics to be sold without prescription. Usually they were added during manufacture of the feed that was then sold at farm dispensaries as a premixed food.

From this time into the 1950s, other antibiotics were tried as growth enhancers by supplementing the animals' feed with small amounts of drugs. Soon penicillin joined chlortetracycline to become one of the two major drugs used as feed additives for cattle, swine, and poultry. Today, many other antibiotics and chemicals have been developed for growth promotion. But penicillins and tetracyclines remain two of the most widely used antibiotics today for this purpose in the United States.

Any therapeutic dose may be 10–100 times greater than a dose used in growth promotion. Treatment is directed against a particular infecting microorganism and the goal is to eradicate or control it as quickly as possible. Given the financial constraints of animal husbandry, money is not wasted and the goal is to use these agents for only as long a time as is necessary to rid the animals of infection. Contagious spread of disease can be fast in large herds. This aim is not very different from a doctor's use of antibiotics to treat humans. But herein lies a significant difference between therapeutic and subtherapeutic use. It is not only the quantity but also the total time of usage that is different.

In the case of growth promotion, smaller doses are administered for longer periods of time, for weeks to months. The net result is that as much as 80% of the total amount of antibiotics given yearly to many food animals goes for growth promotion. We are speaking about 15–17 million pounds of antibiotics used subtherapeutically each year in the United States alone. Antibiotics are provided for growth promotion in other countries as well.

From the data we discussed before, we can estimate that 30 times more animals are being given antibiotics yearly than are humans. Consider with this number the fact that daily animal fecal excretion can be 5–400 times greater than that of humans. For example, the amount of feces excreted by a cow per day is 100 times more than that of a human each day. If an animal is given an antibiotic, the fecal bacteria that survive the antibiotic treatment are resistant to it. Hence, via their excrement, animals are contributing a large amount of resistant bacteria to the natural environment, much larger amounts than are people. The bacteria in this environment move to new areas and new hosts by many routes, through contact with other animals and insects, as well as from food produce.

Growth promotion enthusiasts in the 1950s asked how these drugs actually caused increased growth. Despite some research into the question, the mechanism of action is still not known today. It may be that even small amounts of antibiotics suppress the growth of certain bacteria that compete for needed nutrients. Or, the antibiotics may eliminate those bacteria that suppress the growth of other intestinal strains that are generating the beneficial nutrients for the animals. Some still attribute a hidden nutritional value to antibiotics, although no one has shown that the animals can metabolize them for energy. In most instances, the drugs pass through the animals' intestines unchanged. Against a nutritional mechanism of action is the finding that small doses of antibiotics given to laboratory-housed "germ-free" animals do not show a growth promotion effect. These findings strongly imply that bacteria are somehow involved, either as metabolizers (although this is unlikely), or, more likely, as intestinal competitors for nutrients that are suppressed or eliminated by the antibiotic.

Since bacteria must colonize the intestinal tract in order to survive, one plausible explanation is that low levels of antibiotics are inhibiting the production of proteins involved in adhesion and colonization of the intestinal tract. In this way, certain strains that interfere with the animal's ability to gain the full nutritional value of the feed may be eliminated. These bacteria are, therefore, passed out of the intestinal tract with the feces. It is also possible, especially when husbandry sanitation conditions were less stringent than they are today, that these low doses were suppressing disease by inhibiting infecting bacteria during stressful periods.

What was originally viewed as a boon to animal husbandry, and certainly was in its time, has stirred heated controversy in the United States since the 1970s. From the beginning, unprescribed, over-the-counter use of these valuable agents was frowned upon. It seemed unwise to saturate animals continuously with low doses of the same antibiotics needed to treat their diseases. But the initial reports were glowing: animals did not show allergic reactions; people were not knowingly picking up the antibiotic in their food. Surprisingly, resistant strains of bacteria were reportedly not emerging; however, it is apparent that resistance in bacteria was developing from the beginning but remained undetected. Today, resistance is clearly evident. In fact, wherever food animals are being raised, the bacteria in their intestines and on their skins are largely resistant, not to one antibiotic, but to many different types of antibiotics.

Until 1970, growth promotion usage existed in England and other parts of Europe. Then, a committee of British government-appointed microbiologists and physicians investigated the practice and issued a document that concluded that this practice was harmful to human health. They showed that subtherapeutic doses for prolonged periods produced a strong selection for resistant bacteria in the animal intestinal flora. They reasoned that these bacteria have a potential human risk. And there were instances where some bacteria, namely *Salmonella*, were traced from the animals to disease in people. Since that time, subtherapeutic use of human antimicrobial drugs has been banned in England, a policy that has been followed in other European countries and Canada as well. Other antibacterial agents, not used in human medicine, are being used for growth promotion there.

No such legislative ban has been issued in the United States. What is being asked for in the United States is evidence showing a definite link between antibiotic-resistant bacteria that cause human disease and the use of penicillins and tetracyclines for growth promotion in animals. This is not an easy task because these same drugs are used to treat humans and animals; therefore, selection of the resistant bacteria has potentially resulted from either type of usage. New data, however, are coming closer to providing this information. Several studies have traced resistant infections in humans to the same bacteria in animals and animal food products. Subtherapeutic use was implicated in at least one occurrence of resistant infections, specifically in the spread of *Salmonella* from hamburger meat to people living in four western states in the 1980s.

Notwithstanding the problems caused by the selection of resistant bacteria, the use of antibiotics for growth promotion appears to be having a diminished effect on the animals. More penicillin and tetracycline are now needed to elicit the same increased growth rates they produced in the past. For example, in the 1950s, 5–10 parts per million of tetracycline were effective; today 50–200 parts per million are needed. The dosage is dependent on the kind of animal and the type of antibiotic being used. The trend seems to indicate that growth promotion doses of these antibiotics are gradually reaching the levels recommended for prevention and therapy. Even with the use of higher amounts of antibiotics, the benefits of growth promotion from this usage are less now than those reported twenty years ago. Today, this small growth benefit must be weighed against the environmental and health hazards of a massive selection of resistant bacteria that is a consequence of prolonged antibiotic usage.

Many public interest groups and medical scientists have petitioned the Food and Drug Administration to ban growth-promoting antibiotic usage, notably those involving human therapeutic drugs. Of particular concern are tetracyclines, which affect a large variety of bacteria and select for resistance to themselves and to other antibiotics. Even low doses of the drug select resistant strains of bacteria, and these strains specify high levels of resistance. Besides the spread of the resistant bacteria among animals and from animals to humans, the resistance determinants can be disseminated via transposons or transferable plasmids to other bacteria that colonize people. In fact, the mobile DNA elements found in bacteria in animals are the very same ones found in human strains of the same bacteria.

Animals and humans share in a large, interactive pool of susceptible and resistant bacteria containing movable resistance determinants (Figure 6.1). Humans can pick up these resistant bacteria and resistance genes from animals in different ways. Farm workers can do so during everyday activities in contact with the animals. Consumers do so by eating contaminated foods, especially those that are uncooked. A common scenario is the cook who uses the same kitchen counter to cut and season the meat and prepare the salads. While bacteria on the meat are killed during cooking, the salad retains the bacterial contamination and can even generate increased bacterial numbers if left to sit over a period of time.

Pickup of resistance genes and bacteria from animals can occur indirectly through the use of animal manure as fertilizer. The resistant bacteria in the feces are tilled into the soil or sprayed onto the field. There they multiply and are retained during the harvest. Despite washing, these and other bacteria remain attached to the food crop and enter the consumer's kitchen. One Dutch study followed bacteria from animals to the food chain, then into people, and finally to the sewers.

Farm workers who are in contact with animals have high levels of resistant bacteria in their normal intestinal flora. These resistant strains may have come from animals or may have been

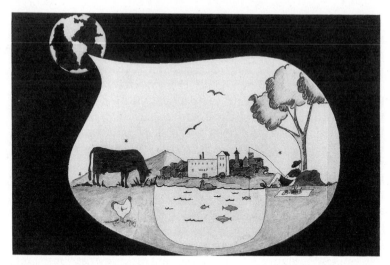

Figure 6.1. This rendition of a quiet environmental scene belies the extensive activity going on at the microscopic level. In fact, bacteria and other microorganisms are multiplying, metabolizing, and exchanging genes. Transfer of bacterial hosts, their plasmids, and genes is occurring among all participants of interactive environments throughout the world, including people, animals, fish, birds, insects, and plants (Bonnie Marshall, Tufts University School of Medicine).

selected and propagated by the antibiotic being used. Bacteria can enter the human body through the mouth, nose, or throat and are swallowed, thus gaining access to the intestinal tract. While some of the bacteria harbored by animals will not colonize humans, it has been documented that a good number can and will. Since we are speaking of normal harmless intestinal bacteria, the presence of resistance is of no immediate concern for farm workers. Moreover, there is no evidence that these workers have more disease than their counterparts working without antibiotics.

The issue is not disease incidence but disease treatment. There are examples of farm workers or their families coming down with diseases that are hard to treat because of antibiotic resistance. This is obvious if the microorganism causes disease. For instance, one outbreak of resistant salmonellosis in a hospital newborn nursery in Connecticut in 1976 was traced to an infected calf on a nearby farm. The mother of the first infected infant came from that farm and was the presumed human source of the nursery infection.

Several experimental studies have brought to light some important facts relating to animal–human bacterial exchange. In the mid-1970s, my laboratory group examined the effect of subtherapeutic levels of a tetracycline antibiotic when introduced into a farm environment. We began with 300 chickens, just hatched from their eggs, that were delivered to a farm in Sherborn, Massachusetts. After initial rearing with heat lamps and a protective covering (Figure 6.2A), the month-old chickens were divided and placed into six different cages for the experiment. Four cages were kept inside a barn; two were placed outside. About 50 chickens were placed in each cage, with males and females equally represented (Figure 6.2B).

One half of the chickens received feed containing subtherapeutic amounts (200 g/ton) of the antibiotic oxytetracycline. Over the course of nine months, we examined the feces of the oxytetracycline-fed and control groups of chickens, as well as the farm workers and family living in the farmhouse about 200 feet away. We also enlisted the help of neighboring families whose children attended the same schools. These people provided weekly stool samples for analysis. They acted as controls for any changes in bacterial flora not attributable to the chickens that might occur over the time period being examined.

Within 24–36 hours of feeding the oxytetracycline-laced feed to the chickens, their intestinal *Escherichia coli* were converted from susceptible to those that were mostly resistant to tetracycline. Over the ensuing three months, other changes occurred. *E. coli* began to appear with resistance not only to tetracycline, but also to ampicillin, streptomycin, and sulfonamides, even though the chickens had never been fed these drugs. In fact, no one had used these drugs on the farm at all.

Gradually, after five to six months, increased resistance appeared in the intestinal *E. coli* of the farm family members. One-

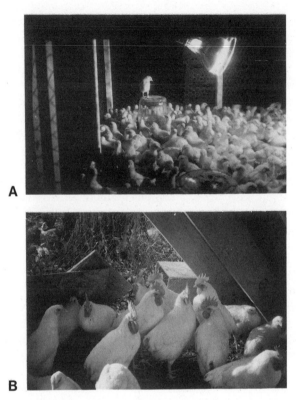

Figure 6.2. A) Newly hatched chickens were reared under heat lamps during the first weeks of life. B) Fifty adult chickens were placed in cages with equal numbers of males and females. The chickens in half the cages were fed with oxytetracycline-supplemented feed; the other half received normal feed.

third of the weekly fecal samples showed an almost complete resistance to tetracycline. Moreover, by the sixth month, the *E. coli* were found to be resistant to four to five different antibiotics. The same phenomenon of multiple resistance that appeared in the chickens appeared to be emerging in the flora of farm inhabitants, even though the people were *not* taking the tetracycline, nor were they eating the chickens. The intestinal flora of their neighbors, the control group, had none of these changes.

The study showed clearly that these relatively small amounts of antibiotic could change the intestinal flora of animals and, more surprisingly, the flora of people living on the same farm. Moreover, chronic use of the drug (for two to three months) led to the emergence of bacteria with resistance to more than one antibiotic.

This appearance of multiple resistance from ingesting a single antibiotic is not unique to this study, or to chickens. It has been observed in other animals and in humans taking a single antibiotic for long periods of time. As noted earlier, women being treated with tetracycline for weeks for urinary tract infections were found to harbor bacteria in their intestines with resistance to many different antibiotics besides tetracycline. Patients taking long-term tetracycline or erythromycin to control acne were shown to harbor many different types of skin bacteria, all bearing resistance to three to six different antibiotics. In all cases, the emergence of multiple resistance followed chronic usage of only one antibiotic. In terms of selection of resistance, there lies one of the crucial differences between therapeutic and subtherapeutic use—the length of usage influences the environmental effect. Chronic use leads to multidrug resistance.

A group of studies during the mid- to late-1980s among pigs on farms in East Germany provided a different insight into the consequences of antibiotic use in animals and, in particular, to the spread of resistance. In this case, the transfer of a resistance determinant was documented from animals to a whole neighboring human population.

The investigators introduced a previously unused antibiotic, streptothricin, into the pigs' feed at levels intended for growth promotion. Before its introduction, no resistance to the drug could be found among bacteria associated with animals and humans, despite careful and quantitative measurements of fecal flora. Within six months of usage, however, a new resistance gene was discovered on transferable plasmids in the intestinal bacteria of the pigs. Of further importance, this resistance determinant was on a transposon, which explained why the resistance gene could be found on plasmids of various types in different intestinal bacteria.

Within two years, this resistance gene was recovered in 16–18% of all *E. coli* isolated from the feces of farm workers and their families as well as among people in the geographic area of the treated pigs. It also appeared in 1% of the bacteria causing urinary tract infections in this area. No streptothricin resistance was observed in people or animals in control areas where the antibiotic was not being used.

This rapid selection and spread revealed the extent of interaction between animal and human ecosystems. It clearly showed that a resistance gene, selected in animals, entered human strains of *E. coli* and even into strains causing human disease. Again, we are not saying that the bacteria are more infectious or will cause more disease. Our point here is that a resistance gene selected in animals can find its way into strains associated with humans. If it happened for the relatively unimportant streptothricin resistance gene, it could happen with others, such as those for resistance to penicillin, tetracyclines, and other human therapeutics. From an *E. coli* host, the resistance gene could eventually end up in bacteria causing disease.

Recently, Bonnie Marshall and other associates in my laboratory examined the natural spread of a resistant *E. coli* from one kind of animal to others and eventually to humans. The experiment was designed to determine if *E. coli* harbored by one animal were somehow naturally confined to that animal. In other words, were there different kinds of *E. coli*, each specific to a particular kind of animal? We isolated an *E. coli* from a calf, marked it in the laboratory so that we could track it in the environment, and gave it back to the calf. The *E. coli* easily colonized the original calf, moved to mice in the same pen, then to pigs, chickens, flies, and wild turkeys—all at significant distances away (Figure 6.3). Human caretakers also began excreting these "calf" *E. coli*. The same phenomenon occurred with *E. coli* taken from pigs. The conclusion was clear. *E. coli* can colonize the intestines of many different kinds of animals. Therefore, there is no safeguard in the fact that

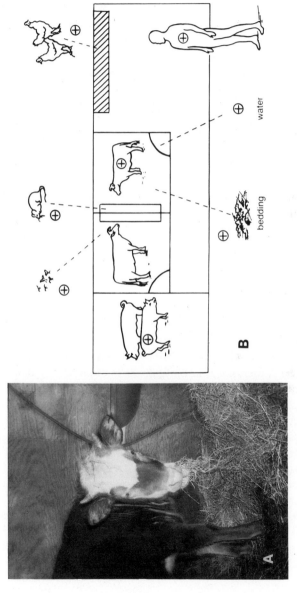

Figure 6.3. Spread of *E. coli* from an inoculated calf on a farm. An *E. coli* from the calf (A) was marked biochemically in the laboratory and refed to the animal. Over time, the "marked" *E. coli* could be recovered from other animate and inanimate objects in the barn (B) (Bonnie Marshall, Tufts University School of Medicine).

the resistant bacteria selected by animal use of antibiotics emerge in the animals. These *E. coli* are environmental; their hosts may be many different animals—including humans.

Transfer can occur in the opposite direction, as well, that is from humans to animals. In a study among baboons in Amboseli National Park in Kenya in 1982, investigators found significantly greater numbers of resistant bacteria in those animals eating human refuse from nearby campers than in their counterparts who lived on the natural diet in the wild (Figure 6.4). On examination of the fecal flora, the animals feeding on human garbage had a flora strikingly similar to humans—diverse numbers of different *E. coli* with various sized plasmids. In contrast, baboons from the wild had flora showing a more harmonious group of *E. coli*, and only a small number of plasmids.

ANIMAL-TO-HUMAN SPREAD OF DISEASE-CAUSING RESISTANT BACTERIA THROUGH FOOD

In the last decade, bacterial contamination of food in the United States has caused sickness, hospitalizations, and even deaths. The infectious microorganism in most cases has been *Salmonella*, a microorganism that causes severe diarrhea. If the bacteria get into the bloodstream and multiply, they cause septicemia characterized by high fevers and often death.

Salmonella is a common infectious agent in animals but can often be carried by the animal as a low-grade or hidden infection. In the past decade, the number of outbreaks of *Salmonella* infections has increased. Moreover, while *Salmonella* strains were uniformly susceptible to antibiotics prior to 1970, recent problems have been caused by *Salmonella* that are resistant to at least two, if not four or five, different antibiotics. In 1981, an outbreak of salmonellosis traced to one brand of precooked roast beef occurred in New Jersey and Pennsylvania and involved about one

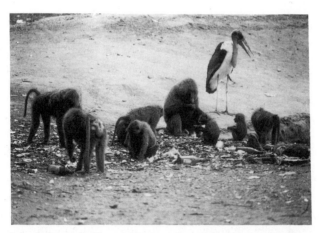

Figure 6.4.   Baboons feeding on human refuse placed in pits near campsites in Amboseli Park in Kenya. These baboons had a higher frequency of antibiotic resistance in their fecal flora than did their counterparts living in the wild.

hundred people who contracted severe diarrhea. The microorganism was multiply resistant.

Investigations by members of the Centers for Disease Control in Atlanta, Georgia showed that such outbreaks caused by multiresistant *Salmonella* are increasing. Significantly, antibiotic ingestion by people is an important contributing factor to this increase. If infecting *Salmonella* are resistant, the chance of infection is higher in the people eating the contaminated product if they are also taking antibiotics to which the *Salmonella* are insensitive. The resistant strain has an advantage when antibiotics are present and smaller numbers are sufficient to take hold in the body and cause disease. Other people, who are not taking an antibiotic but are eating the same contaminated product, might never get the disease because the numbers of infecting bacteria are too low. Had contaminating *Salmonella* microorganisms been susceptible to the antibiotic, this selection would not have taken place.

Another study in 1983, from the Centers for Disease Control, traced a *Salmonella newport* outbreak in four Midwestern states to hamburger meat made from cattle from a single farm. Epidemiologic data showed that 12 of the 18 stricken individuals had been taking antibiotics to which the microorganism was resistant. The first thought of the CDC workers was that the antibiotic preparation was contaminated but, in fact, the antibiotic source of each individual had been different. What was common to each patient was that they had all eaten hamburger meat in the week before they got sick. This meat was traced to beef cattle from one farm in South Dakota adjoining a farm where a *Salmonella* of the same type had been isolated. The *Salmonella* were the same, not only by type, but also by the particular multiresistance plasmid that they contained. Putting the pieces of the puzzle together, the CDC epidemiologists concluded that the likely route of infection was from beef cattle to the meat in processing plants, to the packages in the grocery stores. Again, the concentration of *Salmonella* in the meat was assessed to have been small; hence, many people who ate the hamburger meat were unaffected. Those who were taking antibiotics to which the *Salmonella* were resistant, however, provided a perfect environment for the resistant strain to multiply, leading to overt clinical disease.

In 1985 in California, several hundred individuals who developed diarrhea had *Salmonella newport* isolated from their diarrheal specimens. The source for all these individuals was again hamburger meat. Two people died. The investigators traced the microorganism, identified by its plasmid, to dairy cattle where it could still be isolated. The microorganism was also found in the processing plants and in the remaining unsold meat. Besides using therapeutic antibiotics, the farmer was also feeding subtherapeutic amounts of penicillin and tetracycline to the animals. The *Salmonella* were resistant to the subtherapeutic and therapeutic drugs used on that farm. This was the first definitive study, using biochemical and microbiological techniques, that traced the causative microorganism from an animal source to humans via all parts of the food chain.

Milk has also been a source of *Salmonella* infections. One

outbreak in 1987 in Arizona occurred from raw milk and was traced back to infected animals. One of the largest outbreaks of *Salmonella* infection linked to milk occurred in northern Illinois in the spring of 1985 and affected people in three other states. A total of 200,000 people contracted the disease from packaged milk. Again, studies showed that the antibacterial resistance of the strain increased its attack rate, since, among the infected people, a larger than normal percentage was taking an antibiotic for some reason. This antibiotic ingestion put them at greater risk. Again, the culprit microorganism was multiresistant. The milk, two different brands of pasteurized 2% milk from a single dairy, became contaminated apparently through a leakage in the system that mixed raw milk with pasteurized milk.

These studies should leave no question that domestic animals can be a source of resistant bacterial infections in humans. Since food animals are routinely and chronically being fed antibiotics, the microorganisms that they harbor are often multiply resistant, a situation that produces an additional health hazard to the human population. Paradoxically, being multiresistant, the bacteria pose a greater potential problem to those *already* taking an antibiotic for another illness. While there is less use of antibiotics for growth promotion in the cattle industry than in the swine industry, the beef industry has been the most common source of resistant infections. This is largely because many people's tastes demand rare beef, and the cooking does not kill all the bacteria associated with the raw meat. Only infrequently does meat other than beef get ground up for hamburger, mixing the exposed outer surfaces with the inner tissues. Swine and poultry are generally well cooked, thus killing off any contaminating bacteria.

We may wonder how the subtherapeutic use of drugs can still work effectively. Given the years of usage, one would expect that the antibiotic has selected countless resistant strains. We may also wonder which drugs can be used effectively when these animals get sick.

There are indications that resistance *has* become a problem when trying to treat animals that have been taking subtherapeutic amounts of antibiotics. New drugs are being used to treat illnesses in these animals previously controlled by the older line of antibiotics. Resistance was presumably the reason that the farmer caring for the dairy cows on the farm in California where subtherapeutic doses of penicillin and tetracycline were given, had to use the restricted and illegal antibiotic chloramphenicol to treat his sick cows. The other appropriate antibiotics were useless in the face of resistance. Even in this case, chloramphenicol was ineffective, since these *Salmonella* also bore resistance to the drug—a resistance seen infrequently in clinical strains of bacteria in the United States.

What can be done and what should be done? Many farmers believe that they need these antibiotics in order to raise healthy and hardy animals. This may or may not be true, depending on how the animals are raised and the conditions of the farm, as well as the number of animals being housed together. Certainly, the close confinement practices of some large farm complexes set the stage for cross-contamination with infectious diseases. This is presumably the reason why, in the raising of veal cattle, the milk fed to them is almost uniformly supplemented with tetracycline.

Even though any proposed legislative action to eliminate subtherapeutic use of antibiotics in animal feeds has been delayed in Congress for over fifteen years, the situation is not completely dormant. There is increasing pressure from individuals and public interest groups to limit this type of usage. Mounting evidence has revealed the resistance problem. There is a growing understanding that these valuable human antibiotics are not needed or even useful for promoting growth of animals. The poultry industry, which once used penicillins and tetracyclines universally for growth promotion, claims that only about 20% or less of producers do so now.

Following public concern about the problem of resistant salmonellosis traced to beef, the Cattlemen's Association advised its constituents to stop using antibiotics for growth promotion of beef cattle. They asked that drugs not used in humans, ones other than antibiotics, be the only ones added to the animal feed. Today, this practice is largely followed. Monensin, an animal-use-only chemical, is a successful alternative. So far, however, no changes have been advocated by the swine industry.

New and old alternatives for penicillins and tetracyclines are available for growth promotion. Bacitracins, which are nonabsorbable antibiotics not used for internal human infections but only for local skin lesions, were shown, even in the early 1950s, to produce a growth promotion effect. Some of the early data showed that bacitracin had an effect equal to that of tetracycline. Today bacitracins continue to be used successfully in animal husbandry. In the chicken industry, bacitracins or the bambermycins, another group of nonabsorbable antimicrobials, are the growth promoting agents principally used. This change is a major step forward.

The veterinary profession itself has seen the problems and discrepancies between the availability of antibiotics to livestock owners and the availability to humans. Summarizing their view of veterinary medicine in the 21st century, William Pritchard and Frank Loew described the freer access of animal owners than of laypeople to a multitude of potent antimicrobials. This is also true of livestock owners as compared to pet owners. They estimate that "approximately 93% of the drugs approved for animals can be used by livestock owners without veterinary supervision."[1] They see the public's concern about the "environmental issues raised by these practices and by the potential for contamination of foods with residues and pathogens." They suggest that veterinarians should play active roles in finding the way to reduce the "risks entailed with such widespread use of potent antimicrobials." Veterinarians are certainly an important group to rally for action.

The outcry from animal rights groups about the crowded conditions for raising animals, and the concern shown by microbiologists and clinicians about emergent resistant strains have led to renewed interest in raising animals in the traditional way. "Natural food farms" have begun to proliferate in New York State and in many parts of the Midwest. These farms claim to produce an excellent product without reliance on chemical or antibiotic food additives. The Chicago-based Food Animal Concerns Trust

(FACT), a nonprofit, privately financed organization supports farms that raise animals under conditions where antibiotic supplementation is not given. The group supported the Rambling Rose brand of veal for some time. This veal was produced from nonanemic calves raised outdoors and fed nonantibiotic supplemented milk containing iron and nutrients. Farms were located in New York, Pennsylvania, and Texas. While the meat was dark and not white like that of the anemic calf, a small but sustained market for the product appeared because of the meat's good taste and quality. Some of the finer restaurants in New York, Chicago, and San Francisco boasted the Rambling Rose mark on their menus, including Chanterelle in New York. Because of problems in distribution, this project was discontinued, but the experiment was successful in showing that it could be done and that the product had a market.

Several years ago, FACT launched its first chicken egg product, called Nest Eggs, which was sold throughout the New York, northern New Jersey, and Chicago areas. The hens are raised on farms in Illinois and New Jersey where they are free to roam in straw litter, not crowded in cages. FACT has shown that this alternative measure for raising animals is profitable and successful.

Groups such as the National Resources Defense Council have attempted legal action to get the United States Food and Drug Administration Center for Veterinary Medicine to ban the use of human antibiotics in animal feeds. The efforts have not been legislatively successful but have brought the issues to the public where consumers are heeding the call.

Thus, the combined efforts of livestock owners, veterinarians, and consumers may lead to a change in the use of human therapeutics as growth enhancers in large livestock production. If consumers hold out for more naturally raised products, the producers will inevitably deliver it. Given legislative politics, better-educated consumers will demand animals free of human antibiotic consumption. Only then will we see definitive changes in this area of antibiotic usage.

Chapter 7

FURTHER ECOLOGIC CONSIDERATIONS

Antibiotic Use in Agriculture, Aquaculture, Pets, and Minor Animal Species

The bulk of antibiotics produced in the United States is consumed in the treatment of humans and to promote growth and control infections in food animals. Many of the same drugs, however, have found their places in the treatment of diseases affecting pets, such as dogs and cats, as well as trees, plants, fish, and even honey bees.

Poultry, cattle, and pigs represent the largest group of animals being raised for food consumption, members of what the United States Food and Drug Administration calls the "major species" of animals, which also includes horses, dogs, and cats. Other food animals raised in lesser numbers, such as lambs, sheep, and goats, which are members of the "minor species," likewise receive antibiotics. So do fish and animals raised for their pelts, such as mink.

Compared with the more than 30 million pounds of antibiotics given annually in the United States to the major food animals and to humans, the total amount of antibiotics given yearly to these other animals and used for agriculture is relatively small. It probably accounts for only about half a million pounds. The impact of this use on the environment, namely in the selection of resistant bacteria, however, may still be considerable as we shall discuss.

ANTIBIOTIC USE IN AGRICULTURE

Bacteria and other microbial agents cause diseases in plants and trees. It is, therefore, not surprising to find that antibiotics can control and treat some of these diseases. To get the antibiotic to each plant or tree, however, broad-scale methods are often needed. Although some antibiotics can be injected into tree trunks, today tree farm owners generally treat by spraying antibiotics onto the affected plants and trees. This approach is used chiefly to control infections known to be present or to prevent ones from entering at a particularly vulnerable growth period. As a result, this mode of drug delivery enlarges the potential ecological consequences of antibiotics since application is to an area, not to a single infected host plant. As with other antibiotic treatments, this use on field crops leads to the killing of susceptible bacteria inhabiting that environment, as well as the pathogens under treatment. In a perverse way, therefore, even though these are comparatively small amounts of antibiotics, they have a potentially significant effect vis-à-vis the selection of resistant bacteria. Depending on the scale of dispersal, this usage can be an important contributor to the emergence of resistance in bacteria sharing the environment with human beings.

Two antibiotics, oxytetracycline and streptomycin, are currently registered in the United States for use in the treatment of diseases of trees and plants. This registration dates back about forty years—to the same decade of the discovery of these drugs and their successful use in humans. Today, in the United States, about 40,000–50,000 pounds of antibiotics are used each year just for the control of bacterial infections of fruit trees. One pound (about 450 grams) is enough antibiotic for one day's treatment of 450 people.

Originally discovered in 1943, streptomycin became popular in treating agricultural plant diseases in 1952. Although used more extensively in the 1950s and 1960s, it still holds its own as a common treatment today. For instance, streptomycin is generally applied to mitigate "soft rot" or "black leg" in potatoes (Figure 7.1). These bacterial diseases cause decay of the growing potato tuber. It is also used for the treatment of "wild fire" or "blue mold" of tobacco plant seed beds. These are also bacterial diseases that begin in breaks in the leaf and end up killing the plants. Likewise, to

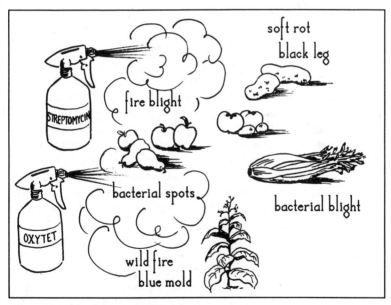

Figure 7.1. Antibiotics, chiefly streptomycin and oxytetracycline, are used to control bacterial infections of fruits and vegetables (Bonnie Marshall, Tufts University School of Medicine).

prevent "bacterial blight" on celery during the transplanting of seedlings, and to protect peppers and tomatoes from "bacterial spot," streptomycin has become a standard treatment.

Oxytetracycline is a form of the more commonly used tetracycline. It is less easily absorbed into the human body and for this reason, has found its place in treating surfaces of animals and plants where absorption into the body is not needed for its activity. For instance, this form of tetracycline is used to treat bacteria in the intestinal tracts of food animals. It is also effective when injected into certain tree roots or trunks to treat bacterial infection.

The species of bacteria that cause diseases in animals and plants are different from those causing infections in man. These bacteria have features similar to bacteria that cause diseases in humans, however, and may be distantly related. They belong to common *families* consisting of multiple types or species that share certain characteristics, although each of the members may show a propensity to infect different human, animal, or plant hosts. For instance, many bacterial agents of plant diseases are classified as mycoplasma or mycoplasmalike. The plant mycoplasma is different from the *Mycoplasma pneumoniae* that causes respiratory tract infections in humans, but they share certain likenesses. They are bacteria that do not have complete cell walls nor the capacity to synthesize them. Because of this feature, they are naturally resistant to antibiotics that affect cell wall synthesis, such as penicillins, but are sensitive to those that affect protein synthesis, such as tetracycline, chloramphenicol, and erythromycin. While not known, it is possible that genetic material, such as resistance genes, could be exchanged between the plant and animal mycoplasma. While only distantly related, the similarities between these kinds of bacteria affecting animals and plants may still be more than that shared by Gram-positive and Gram-negative bacteria known to exchange resistance genes.

Erwinia is a primary target group for antibiotics in the treatment of fruit tree diseases. Members of this genus belong to the Enterobacteriaceae, the same family that includes *Escherichia coli*, *Salmonella*, and *Shigella*. Bacteria in this family can exchange genes among themselves, including plant pathogens. Apple and pear trees are the most important victims of *Erwinia*. *Erwinia amylovora* causes a disease known as "fire blight"—a withering of the leaves and decaying of fruit. The microorganism enters the trees through wounds in the flower or leaf and then moves to other parts of the tree. Streptomycin appears to be the drug of choice in combatting *Erwinia*. In certain areas, however, resistance to streptomycin has appeared in *Erwinia* making streptomycin ineffective. This event has necessitated a change to oxytetracycline, which is, fortunately, effective. Oxytetracycline is likewise efficient in controlling blemishes, or "bacterial spots," on peaches caused by another Gram-negative bacteria, *Xanthomonas*. Applications are generally done by airblast spraying from movable apparatuses pulled by trucks through the rows of trees.

The application of antibiotics to fruit trees occurs throughout the United States, but chiefly on the two coasts. In the western coastal states of Washington, Oregon, and California, primarily pear trees are treated, while antibiotic treatment in the East involves mostly peach and apple trees. Antibiotic application usually begins at the first suspicion or sign of a disease problem.

At the end of the last decade, principally nine states were using oxytetracycline on their fruit trees: New Jersey, Maryland, North Carolina, South Carolina, Georgia, Missouri, Michigan, Illinois, and Indiana. Of the total acreage devoted to growing pear and peach trees in the United States at that time, about 25–30% of the pear crop areas, occupying some 20,000 acres, and 15%, about 15,000 acres, of the peach areas received treatments. Today, the situation is similar. This is not much, considering the vast size of the United States, but could produce significant changes in the bacterial flora of these treatment sites and the people living there.

Aerial spraying by airblasts from the ground and occasionally by airplanes (this latter method having declined in recent years) results in antibiotic application to areas outside those specified for treatment. Dusting, such as on potatoes, and hand-held sprayers allow homeowners and gardeners to treat their own plants and fruit trees with a greater degree of confinement. Both applications, however, potentially affect more than the immediate environment. With dusting, the user's own intestinal and skin flora may be "treated," since small amounts of antibiotics can be ingested or deposited on the skin.

Antibiotics are applied on other types of vegetation besides fruit trees. Antibiotics exert a beneficial effect by delaying or controlling "lethal yellowing," a mycoplasmalike infection of ornamental palms, coconut palms, date palms, and others. In the 1970s in Miami, 40,000 coconut palms were affected, killing 75% of those in Dade County. Oxytetracycline by injection is the drug of choice for the problem and is used mainly in Florida and Texas.

Among ornamental plants, chrysanthemums are treated by placing cuttings directly into an antibiotic solution in order to protect them against bacterial diseases. Dieffenbacchia, philodendron, and pyracantha are often treated with antibiotics for bacterial diseases that lead to withering of the leaves, or so-called "fire blight." As in all plant applications, the aim of treatment is prevention, since no cure is attainable in plants once they become diseased. Therefore, it is important for the grower to know exactly when during growth these plants are most likely to contract disease.

During the 1950s, when streptomycin was being used on fruit trees, the United States Food and Drug Administration examined the fruit for residues. Within the limits of detection (0.5 parts per million), no residues were found. This examination is still done periodically wherever treatments are applied, to assure that no residual antibiotic can be inadvertently ingested by the consumer. This safeguard is important; however, the long-term effect on the microbial ecology of an agricultural area, that is, the selection of resistant strains of bacteria, cannot be monitored so easily.

Although streptomycin is one of the two most popular antibiotics used on plants, it is rarely used today in human medicine because of the discovery of newer and less toxic agents. Streptomycin resistance, for some unknown reason, is among the most common resistances found in bacterial strains associated with humans. However, some believe this is the result of prior streptomycin selection followed by continued propagation, despite the absence of the antibiotic. Curiously, streptomycin resistance rarely occurs alone; it is generally found in conjunction with other resistance determinants. Therefore, while streptomycin resistance per se may have little consequence on human therapy today, when streptomycin is used, it selects not only bacteria with streptomycin resistance but also those bearing resistance to other useful antibiotics. In this way, the environmental pool of multiresistance is widened. Certain *Erwinia amylovora* have been isolated with multidrug resistance on transferable plasmids. From the standpoint of agriculture, streptomycin or tetracycline resistance, when it occurs, seriously thwarts plant therapy, since few approved alternative antibiotics are available.

The heyday of antibiotic treatment of plants and trees was in the 1950s during the height of antibiotic discovery. But as time passed, the disease-causing microorganisms began to appear to be resistant to the very drugs being used to kill them—just as we have seen in the treatment of humans. Clinicians, microbiologists, and veterinarians also began to raise health concerns about the residues left on food produce. In response to these concerns, other means of disease control, such as nonantibiotic chemical treatments, began to replace the use of antibiotics. Not all substitute measures, however, could supplant antibiotics. Some disease agents could not be managed any other way. Therefore, streptomycin and oxytetracycline are still important agents in treating certain susceptible bacterial diseases of fruit and agricultural crops. Guarding the susceptibility of this population must be a goal, given the already high frequency of resistance to these antibiotics in other bacteria in the environment. As in other areas, therefore, misuse and particularly prolonged use should be avoided.

The major problem we are addressing here is not antibiotic residues on or in food produce but rather the enormous selection that even small amounts of these agents can have for resistant bacteria. In the wake of killing susceptible bacteria, resistant forms, even rare ones, emerge, propagate, and can predominate in the treated area. There are no present-day tests for measuring the frequency of these resistant bacteria. They could someday be a problem to agriculture. They could also have wider consequences.

If they find their way into the vicinity of bacteria that colonize the gut or the skin of people or animals, they could pass their resistance traits to these bacterial strains. In this way, resistance traits selected in agriculture could be spread to humans.

Contamination of crops with antibiotic-resistant microorganisms of more potential clinical relevance may occur by another route. Resistant fecal strains of bacteria can contaminate agricultural plots and their crops through the use of manure from antibiotic-fed animals. In certain areas of England, Europe, and the United States, conveyer belts move fecal slush from pigs or other animals out to agricultural lands where it is aerated and dispersed as a spray onto the growing agricultural plants. It is through this application that resistant bacteria could be transferred from animals to other ecosystems, in this case agricultural products. Studies have shown that birds feeding amongst the dispersed manure pick up and ingest these resistant microorganisms. Flies can carry fecal *Escherichia coli* for quite long distances. The full extent of this procedure's contribution to the general problem of antibiotic resistance in humans is not yet understood. Given our current situation with the enlarging pool of multiple antibiotic resistances, we should devote time to studying this area of potential antibiotic resistance spread.

How resistant bacteria actually travel through the food chain can be explained through various scenarios. Washing fruits or vegetables may clean off the dirt, but washing can cause a more thorough spread of existing bacteria. If a vegetable has leaves or crevices, bacteria can find their way into these or even into its interior. The outer leaves of lettuce are full of bacteria from the soil and from manure and other contacts with animals and humans. In contrast, the inner leaves are virtually clean. Unless lettuce is washed leaf by leaf, as the French people usually do, the bacteria from the outside leaves enter the inside ones. The removal of the pedicel from a tomato (plucked from the plant) leaves an opening to the inside of the fruit. Thus, bacteria may enter into the tomato where they find plenty of nutrients for growth and multiplication.

In studies of bacteria associated with fruits and vegetables from local food markets in Boston, we have found large numbers, 10,000 to 100,000, of antibiotic-resistant bacteria per gram of vegetable. These bacteria were not particularly harmful, but 10–20% of them were potentially able to colonize human intestines. While they were not disease-causing, these strains did carry resistance genes that could be transferred to other bacteria in laboratory experiments. In immunocompromised patients, such as those undergoing cancer chemotherapy, even these relatively harmless bacteria can result in disease. If resistant, they would be more difficult to treat. For instance, on this market produce we found *Klebsiella* bacteria with multiple resistance on plasmids that were transferable to *Escherichia coli*, a natural member of our intestinal flora. While not usually harmful, *E. coli* becomes a reservoir for resistance traits that could give a person trouble later, especially in an immunocompromised state during cancer therapy. Recall, for example, the previously discussed patient who died from a multi-drug resistant *E. coli* while being treated for leukemia.

I once instructed hospital medical staff, during a learning exercise, to take a tomato, slice it with a sterile knife, and then place the slice for several seconds on top of agar that contained nutrients for growth. After the slice was removed, the plate was incubated overnight at body temperature (37°C or 98°F). The next day the complete image of the tomato slice was replicated on the plate, designed by colonies from the bacteria within the tomato. None of the bacteria were harmful—mostly soil types or those carried by humans and animals in our intestinal tracts. Further study, however, showed that about 10% of these bacteria were antibiotic resistant and, again, were the kinds that could colonize our intestinal tract.

On the basis of these studies and those performed by others elsewhere, uncooked fruits and vegetables are conventionally removed from the diets of patients undergoing therapy for cancer at a time when their host defense systems are suppressed and when common bacteria can take over and cause severe disease.

Antibiotic use in agriculture is varied. The applications are very different from those used in animals and humans. The environmental ramifications from even small doses can still be significant in the selection of resistant variants. Some of these may bear transferable resistance plasmids and transposons, bringing direct problems to the agricultural growers and potential changes to other participants in our shared environment.

ANTIBIOTIC USE IN HONEYBEES

American and European foulbrood diseases cause the death of countless honeybees and consequent loss of hives. In the United States, oxytetracycline is the only antibiotic permitted for use in bee hives. American foulbrood is caused by *Bacillus larvae*, a rod-shaped Gram-positive bacterium; the European disease is caused by *Streptococcus pluton*, a Gram-positive coccus. In general, the antibiotic is recommended only for preventing and controlling the disease from spreading from one infected hive to others in the vicinity of the infected hive. Some beekeepers use this antibiotic for treatment of the infected hive itself, but this application has been vigorously debated. Some states have laws against it. Many believe that treatment of infected hives does not help the overall beehive situation. For one thing, it could lead to resistant bacteria and, thus, cause ineffective treatment if later infections arise. For another, once the bacteria, namely *B. larvae*, are established, it is hard, if not impossible, to get rid of them. Consequently, it is better to destroy the hive with the bacteria. There is also the possibility that infected hives could contain bees that are some- how more susceptible to infectious agents. Therefore, if these bees and their hives are salvaged, the effect would be to propagate hives that are more susceptible, not only to this foulbrood disease, but also to other potential disease-causing agents.

Treatment is usually given in the early spring and fall, when there are few flowers in bloom. At this time, in the absence of nectar sources, the bees pick up the infection by scavenging honey from other infected hives. During those periods of potential infection, oxytetracycline is applied in powdered sugar directly to the hive. It is the larvae that must be protected. The adult bees, in the process of housekeeping, remove the antibiotic sugar mix and thus make contact with the tetracycline. It is then inadvertently delivered by them to their brood of larvae, which, in this way, receive protection from the infectious agents.

Some history of antibiotic use in bees is in order. In the early 1950s, other antibiotics such as sulfathiazole and streptomycin were used to treat foulbrood disease. Because these drugs did not work effectively, however, erythromycin, a different kind of antibiotic, was added. Then in 1955, in San Luis Valley, Colorado, beekeepers noted that the disease was suddenly not responding to erythromycin. This event, and other similar cases elsewhere, were among the first to alert beekeepers to the problem of bacterial resistance. The emergence of antibiotic-resistant bacteria contributed to the decision to destroy infected hives rather than to propagate weak hives and their resistant bacteria.

From the time that oxytetracycline was first introduced, honey was routinely examined for drug residues. None were found. According to an official in the Division of Beneficial Insects Laboratory of the United States Department of Agriculture, the reason is that the antibiotic is not stable, and breaks down in the hive and in honey. This laboratory of the USDA also periodically checks for resistant *Bacillus* from among bacterial isolates sent to them from infected hives. Until now, no oxytetracycline resistance in the bacillus causing this disease has been found. This is indeed fortunate, since other members of the genus *Bacillus* are known to carry resistance to this antibiotic. By the present treatment method, oxytetracycline loses its effectiveness in the hive in less than ten days. Thus, it does not remain as a continued selective agent. This may be a reason for the yet unseen problem of resistance to it. The application of oxytetracycline to control infection of honeybee larvae is not perceived as a particular contributor to environmental selection of antibiotic resistant bacteria. Our interest in describing this practice is to point out how diverse antibiotic usage is as an almost everyday happening. Moreover, it may be that in this limited area, careful use may be controlling a potential resistance problem. Certainly, if resistance should emerge, then preventive use of tetracyclines will have to be changed. Which alternative drugs will be as safe and as effective is unknown. It would be in the best interests of the beekeeper to continue to have tetracycline available as the drug of choice. In order to assure this present situation, the current use of tetracycline must remain appropriate, that is, given only when needed.

ANTIBIOTIC USE IN COMMERCIAL FISH

Many of the antibiotics effective in human medicine are also used for the treatment of bacterial infections in salmon, catfish, trout, and other commercially raised fish. These antibiotics include oxytetracycline, sulfamerazine (a sulfonamide derivative) and ormetoprim (a derivative of trimethoprim). In particular, they are used to treat ulcers or furunculoses of the skin of the fish, as well as diarrhea and blood-borne sepsis. These infections are caused by rodlike Gram-negative microorganisms belonging to bacterial families that also produce disease in humans. To ensure protection of the consumer against antibiotic residues, the United States Food and Drug Administration requires a withdrawal time before fish can be harvested and sold. Withdrawal times depend both on the antibiotic and the fish. For instance, in catfish the withdrawal time for ormetoprim is 3 days, but for salmon it is 42 days. The withdrawal time for oxytetracycline is 21 to 30 days for all fish.

These times of withdrawal before marketing are dependent on the total amount of antibiotic given for treatment and the ability of the antibiotic to remain in the fish once the antibiotic has been discontinued. The timing between withdrawal and sales is based on studies looking at how long residues actually remain in the body of the fish. Ideally, antibiotic treatments of fish are kept to short time periods, thus eliminating the buildup of these drugs in the fish. While the concerns of the consumer regarding antibiotic residues in the fish may be answered by these control measures, the ecologic effects of antibiotic use here are the same as those elsewhere. Furthermore, an increasing number of resistance problems in the treatment of infections in fish is coming to light, as we shall discuss.

The Catfish Industry

About 350 million pounds of catfish are produced annually in the United States and sold on the wholesale market (Figure 7.2). The industry, valued at over $750 million, is centered in the southeastern United States, principally the state of Mississippi, followed by Alabama, Arkansas, Georgia, Florida, and Louisiana.

Catfish ponds vary greatly in terms of size and general farming practices. Farms can be as large as 20–30 acres for the typical commercial pond in the Mississippi Delta or as small as one quarter of an acre on a private farm (Figure 7.2). Commonly the farmer stocks his ponds so that he will have a load of about 5000 fish per acre. In more intensive farming with aeration, the number of fish can reach 8000 per acre. The typical single-family farms may have small ponds, the so-called "mom and pop" ponds, which contain only about 2000 fish per acre. Harvesting in the small farms consists of drainage of the ponds and collection of the fish left in the residual water. This is usually done in the winter. Ponds of large commercial enterprises, generally, are not drained. Most commercial units employ nets that collect only the larger, more mature fish and allow the smaller fish to pass through. They then restock the ponds to achieve the optimum population. The companies add more water to make up for evaporation. These different practices influence the conditions the catfish must endure, the kinds of diseases they might contract, and the ways they might contract them.

Antibiotics enter the scene as soon as disease becomes evi-

A

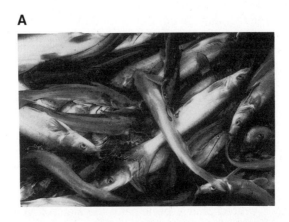

B

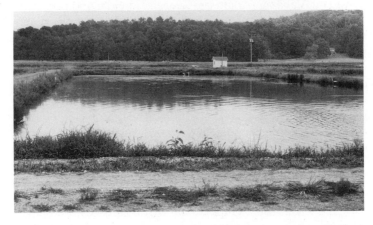

Figure 7.2. A) Catfish recently harvested from a farm in Mississippi (Angelo DePaola, United States Food and Drug Administration, Daulphin Island, Alabama). B) A typical 14-acre catfish pond (Angelo DePaola, United States Food and Drug Administration, Daulphin Island, Alabama).

dent. Whenever dead fish surface, antibiotics are added to the ponds, generally as feed additives (Figure 7.3). The common bacterial diseases, namely those of the skin or blood, are caused by Gram-negative bacteria of the *Aeromonas* and *Edwardsiella* types. Fish are more susceptible to infections at temperatures between 22 and 28°C (72–82°F). Below 28°C, the immune systems of fish are not active, so they are more likely to become diseased; below 22°C bacteria do not survive well, so the fish are protected. Thus, between 22 and 28°C, higher numbers of bacteria are present in the pond and fish have depressed immune systems. Consequently, infection becomes more probable. Such conditions generally occur in the spring and fall. The most popular means of treatment are tetracycline or ormetoprim combined with sulfa-dimethoxine added to the feed or obtained as a premixed medicated feed. The preparation is usually in an oil base so that the antibiotic will not be lost by dissolving into the water or becoming so diluted that the concentrations lose their effectiveness. In

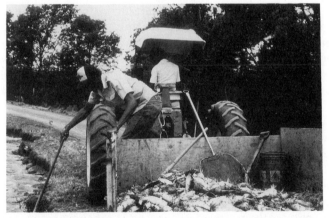

Figure 7.3. Workers collect dead catfish floating on the pond's surface. This occurrence indicates the need for antibacterial therapy (Angelo DePaola, United States Food and Drug Administration, Daulphin Island, Alabama).

general, the tetracycline feeding continues for 10 days with a 21-day withdrawal period. The feeding of ormetoprim and sulfadimethoxine takes place for 5 days with a withdrawal time of 3 days. Ponds that are not completely drained from prior antibiotic treatments may contain considerable amounts of active drug residue after each cycle. Thus, newly introduced fish are subjected to residual antibiotics and to antibiotic-resistant bacteria.

While antibiotic residues in the fish product could be a problem, this possibility is reduced by the withdrawal of the antibiotics before harvest. Another potential adverse effect is not so easily managed, that is, the selection of resistant bacteria that will propagate and could eventually be carried to the consumer on the commercial product.

A common infectious microorganism, *Aeromonas hydrophila*, causes sepsis in catfish and can sometimes lead to diarrhea and sepsis in certain susceptible people who might ingest the microorganisms. In two states, Mississippi and Alabama, 90% of these bacteria associated with the catfish ponds tested resistant to tetracyclines and other antibiotics. As in other instances, the most important consequence of tetracycline resistant bacteria for this industry is the inability to control infections that were once treatable with this relatively inexpensive drug. A further consequence is that these resistant microorganisms can be passed to humans through the food chain. In fact, resistant forms of these bacteria have been found on the carcasses of catfish being sold at market. This finding raises more environmental concern than medical fears, since these bacteria are not particularly infectious to people. The chances of this transfer occurring is minimal once the fish is cooked. "Pickup" of these bacteria, however, can occur on hands during preparation in the home and, thus, they can eventually reach the intestines. The other possible source would be contamination of other foods prepared on the same kitchen surface. Therefore, it is important to wash all foods to be eaten uncooked and to prepare them on surfaces separate from those being used to prepare the raw fish.

The catfish industry continues to expand. At the present time, it is located only in the southeastern states. It is inevitable that this profitable industry will grow in the coming years. As it does, it will use larger and larger total amounts of antibiotics. Eventually the quantity could equal or rival the large amounts of antibiotics used in animal husbandry. This situation will augment the environmental pool of resistant bacteria being selected and propagated in commercial animals.

The Salmon Industry

Salmon farming is another industry that uses considerable amounts of antibiotics, particularly tetracyclines and sulfonamides. United States production is now at 55 million pounds a year. One estimate ascribes 147 pounds of antibiotic applied per acre of salmon per year. These salmon pens are placed in natural sea waters. Therefore, the antibiotics and resultant resistant strains of bacteria created by these farms will have contact with other marine life. As a result, antibiotics used for raising salmon represent another selective force for resistant strains in yet another environmental niche.

Aware of the ecological changes accompanying salmon rearing, notably the contamination of the water beds and other marine life, lobstermen and families in northern Maine fought successfully against the invasion of their area by a Norwegian company wanting to set up a salmon fishery. While companies contend that the antibiotics are used only when needed, it is well known that, because of crowded conditions, antibiotics are required routinely and for long periods of time. Since they are deposited in the water, they can be picked up easily by other marine animals. Tetracycline is not rapidly degraded in fish. Thus, it is excreted in its active state in feces and deposited on the sea floor. Here, too, it remains relatively stable, out of direct sunlight, which can degrade it. Consequently, the ecological effect of this antibacterial agent in the sea is the same as it is in land animals. The long-term selection of resistant and multiresistant bacteria in salmon and other marine life forms not only poses a barrier to the treatment of diseases in the fish themselves, but this selection also provides a means by which these resistance genes can move into the human food chain, either on the fish themselves or through other edible marine animals.

ANTIBIOTIC USE IN MINOR SPECIES OF ANIMALS

Sheep, goats, mink, rabbits, foxes, and other animals raised in small numbers all receive antibiotics at different times in their lives. In fowl, besides the large quantities used in treating or raising chickens and turkeys, antibiotics are also given to pheasants, quail, and ducks. Among the most important antibiotics for these purposes are the tetracyclines, penicillin G, neomycin, streptomycin, and sulfur derivatives. In these animals, as in cattle and pigs, the antibiotics are used most often for growth promotion and to increase the growth efficiency of the feed. Even minks are fed antibiotics in order to increase their pelt sizes.

All preparations are usually given as an additive to the feed, generally at low levels ranging from 20 to 50 grams per ton. Since all the antibiotics are also human therapeutics, they serve as yet another source for selection of resistant bacteria that gain access to the environmental pool shared with man. Of course, the bacterial flora of those people having direct contact with the animals and the antibiotics will receive the greatest impact. But wherever these animals or their products are sent, bacteria can go along with them, thus entering new ecological areas.

ANTIBIOTIC USE IN THE HOME: THE FAMILY PET

About 40% of households in the United States have dogs. In some areas, this number may be as high as 50%. Dogs also carry antibiotic resistant bacteria, as do cats. Studies during the last decade examined the feces from healthy dogs, looking for the frequency of antibiotic-resistant bacteria and transferable resistance determinants. They were present at high frequency. By one study, 65% of almost 100 dogs carried tetracycline-resistant *E. coli*, of which most were multiresistant. Since these pets were not taking antibiotics at the time, the authors suggested that the origin of these resistant bacteria might be commercial dog food or other neighboring animals on antibiotics. Another study taking place in Ireland found that about 70% of the *E. coli* isolates from dogs were multiply resistant. High levels of resistance were also recorded in Australia where 40% of the fecal samples taken from domestic dogs contained multiresistant bacteria. These studies show that already in the 1980s, dogs in diverse geographical areas were harboring relatively high levels of antibiotic-resistant *E. coli* in their fecal flora. These strains represent another environmental constituent capable of exchanging resistance genes.

Besides dogs and cats, for which most antibiotics are given by veterinarian prescription, a variety of antibiotics are readily available over the counter in pet stores throughout the world for smaller animal species. Birds, rodents, and fish are some of the pets for whom these antibiotics can be purchased (Figure 7.4). The drugs are packaged as capsules, tablets, or, occasionally, in liquid or powder forms. Although the total amount of these antibiotics could be considered relatively small compared with that used in animals, humans, and agriculture, their easy availability have potentially unfavorable consequences.

The way that these antibiotics are distributed also raises some important questions and problems. Of particular note, the form and appearance of these drugs are remarkably similar to antibiotics used for treating people. Perhaps this is why some pet store owners and personnel with whom I've spoken have admitted taking these antibiotics occasionally to treat themselves. They perceive these antibiotic pet preparations to be the same as those used in human medicine, and they are available without a doctor's prescription.

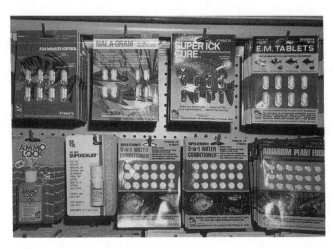

Figure 7.4. Common human therapeutics are offered over the counter for the treatment of small pets, such as fish, rodents, and birds. This is a display of different antibiotic preparations for treating fish.

For instance, each tetracycline capsule for fish contains 250 mg of tetracycline. This is exactly the same formulation sold for human consumption (Figure 7.5). The price of these over-the-counter antibiotics is generally similar to that of those sold by prescription for human use, except that the pet preparations are usually provided in boxes of 8–10 pills. Thus, for some antibiotics, they may actually be cheaper. While scanning the numerous shelves of antibiotics recommended for pets, I was struck by the brilliant colors. Each antibiotic was encased in its own bicolored capsule, some of which resembled color combinations of the same antibiotics sold for human use. The most common antibiotics were the same ones commonly used by people, namely penicillins, tetracyclines, and sulfonamides. Their uses, as indicated on the packages, are for treating obvious signs of disease, such as failure to eat or diarrhea.

The advice for antibiotic treatment generally comes from the

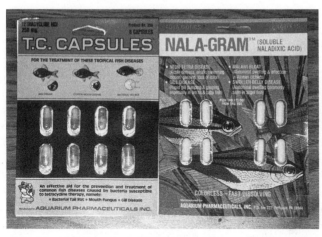

Figure 7.5. Two of the popular antibiotics, tetracycline and nalidixic acid, recommended for pet owners to use for their fish.

pet store owner or worker in response to a query from the pet owner. Jack, the manager of one pet store I visited, explained a common scenario. "A pet owner comes in to me and describes the pet's problems—diarrhea, ruffled feathers, shortness of breath. Based on the kinds of symptoms and descriptions, I prescribe an antibiotic."

When I asked how he made his decisions, he simply answered "based on my own experience." If the pet does not recuperate within the next two days, Jack simply prescribes a second antibiotic. Usually he begins by prescribing one of the tetracycline preparations. If that doesn't work, his second choice is erythromycin.

Jack's familiarity with the antibiotic names was surprising to me, but did not seem particularly unusual to him. I asked if he had a background in pharmacology. "None," he replied, "But I've been in the pet business for a long time."

Jack has worked in this particular store for over ten years, and now manages it. All kinds of pet fish and products for fish are displayed in the more than 1,000 square feet of shelf space. There are other areas furnishing antibiotics and other treatments for birds, rodents, and other small animals. Shelves and tables all around the store display foods and medications for these pets. Jack, with unabashed aplomb, explained the use of antibiotics for the treatment of different pet fish. He saw no problem with the fact that pet owners ask him for advice, and that his initial suggestion is to start with an antibiotic. He sees his role as that of a practitioner giving out all kinds of drugs, including antibiotics. Yet, these are the same antibiotics that require a doctor's prescription when given to humans.

Jack admitted that he has used an antibiotic prepared for fish for himself. He explained that he once had an inflamed finger that was bothering him and looked infected. So, he called a friend of his who is a nurse to ask for some advice. She told him that at the hospital doctors usually treat this kind of problem with erythromycin. So, according to Jack, "I knew that we had human grade erythromycin for fish." He had learned this from the literature he receives with the antibiotic. "It's an antibiotic made under the same conditions as for humans," Jack explained. "So, I went and took it." His finger got better. Jack said that he is not the only one who takes antibiotics meant for pets. At professional meetings he has learned that this is not an unusual practice, nor is it of any great concern to pet store owners and workers.

Jack claimed that he knows which of the antibiotics are human grade and which are not. Although all labels do state "not for human use," the shop owners know that it may be human grade. Jack is aware that those without a human grade designation may not be as pure or sterile and might not be prepared in a way that is guaranteed harmless to people. In general, the nonhuman grade products are those sold in bulk to the pet store owners to use in their resident animals and fish. These include a broad range of antibiotics: tetracycline, erythromycin, sulfur drugs, ampicillin, puromycin, and neomycin.

Our primary concern here is not that antibiotics are being

used for these pets. If they are sick and antibiotics are needed, they should get them. The antibiotics sold, however, are the very ones used currently for humans. More importantly, in contrast to human preparations, these are readily available to pet owners for personal use. Treating the family pet will lead to the same kind of ecological phenomenon that occurs with antibiotic use anywhere, that is, selection of resistant bacteria. While these bacteria may not be infectious for humans, they do add to the environmental pool of resistance genes that can be transferred to bacteria of all kinds, including those associated with people. And in the case of the intestinal *E. coli*, the bacteria can become part of the owners' intestinal flora. Again, we are not advising against this use, only that it be appropriate.

You can buy eight 200 mg capsules of erythromycin for fish for about $4.00, an excellent price by human drug standards. The same antibiotic and newer members of this antibiotic family are enjoying a comeback in human medicine because of their broadened effectiveness against microorganisms causing skin and respiratory diseases. Furthermore, new formulations make the antibiotic less irritable to the gastrointestinal tract. Resistance to erythromycin has emerged in some of the bacteria for which this drug is used in humans. We discussed the current problem surrounding erythromycin-resistant streptococcus in Finland and the association between this finding and increased sales of erythromycin for human use in Finland. We can wonder whether or not resistance problems are emerging in bacteria that cause animal and pet fish diseases. While it has never been shown, there is also the possibility that resistance traits selected in fish bacteria could be transferred to bacteria associated with humans. This scenario is not farfetched, since these kinds of transfers can be detected among bacteria in the laboratory.

These are hypothetical events. What is of known concern is the fact that people visiting pet shops have easy access to therapeutics presently used by humans. These include ampicillin (a modified penicillin with broad antibacterial activity used widely in human medicine), kanamycin (an aminoglycoside used in treating childhood diseases), and nalidixic acid (used in urinary tract infections and certain diarrheas). You may remember that nalidixic acid is the forefather of the newly developing quinolone family of antimicrobial agents with activity against a wide group of bacteria causing urinary tract infections, bone infections, and septicemias. As you learned, resistance to these new drugs is already appearing in bacteria that cause human disease. Whenever these drugs are used for human or nonhuman purposes, resistance traits can be selected; therefore, appropriateness in their applications should be the standard everywhere.

But the problem doesn't end with the easy availability of single agents. An imported group of antibiotics prepared for pet fish consists of preparations with a broad activity range, that is, an effectiveness against many different kinds of bacteria. One of these products contains a combination of antibiotics. Besides the mixing of a sulfonamide and trimethoprim (which is one of the few combinations of antimicrobials used in human medicine), the same medication includes a third antibiotic, called metronidazole, a drug used in treating anaerobic infections. These latter infections are caused by bacteria in the bowel that cannot grow in air. Placing three potent antimicrobials in one medication means that one treatment will distribute three different powerful agents into the immediate environment with the potential to select resistant forms to any one or *all three*.

Another antibiotic formulation for fish has four different antibiotics provided as "flakes" that could be given to fish according to the pet owner's discretion. The decision would be made based on the apparent symptoms of the pet as summarized on the cylindrical container. The top of the container is turned, as for pepper and spices, and out comes the specific flakes of antibiotic wanted. Flake A is chloramphenicol, to be used for cottonlike fluff on mouths and fins, ulcers, and other similar maladies. Flake B, tetracycline, attacks "fin and tail rot." Flake C, dihydrostreptomycin, treats weight loss, fading colors or loss of scales, while Flake D, a combination of metronidazole, sulfadimethoxine, and trimethoprim, is suggested for "introducing new fish," "swollen body," or "swimming on the side."

All these descriptions are expected to be understood easily by the pet fish owner. All these antibiotics have very special uses in human medicine and are rarely, if ever, found together. The kind of decision-making process used in selecting a treatment for fish and other pets may not differ greatly from the kinds of decisions that people are moved to make when seeking medical treatment or when treating themselves. This product labelling exemplifies how real the concept of indiscriminate antibiotic ingestion is to human consumers and how it indirectly challenges the "antibiotic by prescription" rule of human medicine. The relaxed attitude toward using these antibiotics for pets is perhaps reflective of the same attitude toward the use of these drugs in people. If people can give antibiotics to their pets, which many regard almost as dearly as family, why shouldn't they treat themselves or their loved ones? Although neither the pet store industry nor the companies producing these drugs are promoting such an attitude, the real life situation lends itself to such abuses.

In an indirect and subtle way, the respect for antibiotics that we would like to engender in people is undermined by the ready access and self-medication involved in treating household pets. While the quantity of this antibiotic use is small in the scheme of things, these applications are everyday occurrences. We must consider them seriously, at least at some level, in our efforts to preserve a concerned respect toward these irreplaceable drugs.

The examples we have discussed in this chapter further illustrate how ubiquitously antibiotics are used in every aspect of our lives. Therefore, is it any wonder that we have antibiotic resistance? Our point throughout is to be aware of the consequence of this use, since it can bear on the future efficacy of these precious drugs.

Chapter 8

FUTURE PROSPECTS

New Advances against
Potential Disaster

The past decade has seen the unprecedented rise in the spread of antibiotic resistance determinants among disease-causing bacteria. These resistant bacteria have colonized ecological niches in countries worldwide, making all geographic areas vulnerable to the problem of ineffective therapy for bacterial diseases. This situation raises the staggering possibility that a time will come when antibiotics as a mode of therapy will be only a fact of historic interest. While scientific advances may eventually offer a way to replace antibiotics with other means of treating disease, we would rather make that decision ourselves instead of being forced to abandon antibiotic therapies because they have become useless. Despite innovative work on vaccines and other methods of increasing our body's defenses against infection, most scientists and physicians cannot imagine a future without antibiotics.

As for the foreseeable future, I do not envision complete antibiotic failure. Most bacteria are still susceptible to at least some of the antibiotics available currently. The choice of effective antibiotics, however, is growing narrower while new antibiotics are making their way into the marketplace very slowly. We have already reached the point where the cost and availability of particular antibiotics have compromised therapy in certain parts of the world.

Some analysts warn of present-day scenarios in which infectious antibiotic-resistant bacteria devastate whole human populations. They say, "Isn't this already the situation with resistant strains of *Staphylococcus aureus*?" These bacteria, often called "golden staph" because of the gold color of the colonies on laboratory agar, are the scourge of hospitals, where they cause surgical and blood-borne infections characterized by high fevers, sweats, and drops in blood pressure. Death is not uncommon.

In the late 1970s and early 1980s, multiresistant golden staph plagued hospitals in Melbourne, Australia. This situation certainly epitomized the gravest of antibiotic resistance problems. At first insidious and unrecognized, these multiply resistant staphylococci soon became evident as the cause of death among unsuccessfully treated patients in hospitals throughout the Melbourne area. The problem surfaced not just in one hospital, but in many.

The situation raised such havoc and fear that ambulance drivers wore masks to protect themselves from "catching" the golden staph. The concern was not unjustified. Hospital microbiologists and infection control nurses traced the resistant microorganism to hospital personnel and to inanimate objects, including the hospital linens and washing facilities. While this kind of bacteria is always difficult to treat, the Melbourne strain was resistant to all traditional first-line antibiotics. It was also resistant to antiseptics, making this form of cleaning ineffective. Only one antibiotic, vancomycin, remained effective. But this drug was very expensive and also potentially toxic, and, therefore, had to be used sparingly.

The severity of the hospital staphylococcus problem in Melbourne spurred the formation of a local group of hospital personnel who sought to curb and control the spread of the microorganism. They surmised that proper hygiene, notably handwashing among doctors and nurses, and containment of infected patients in designated areas, would help. Additionally, they suggested more judicious use of antibiotics, the source of resistance selection. Out of this group effort came the development and publication of a booklet called *Antibiotic Guidelines*, which explained how to use antibiotics more wisely. Besides producing the book, the developers used innovative ways to publicize it (Figure 8.1).

This critical real life problem formed the core example for a British BBC and American "Nova" TV documentary in 1984, which focused on the global problem of antibiotic resistance. Fortunately,

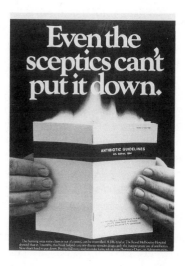 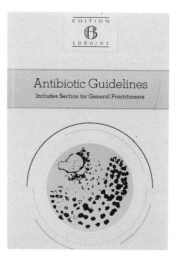

Figure 8.1. Following a massive outbreak of multiresistant *Staphylococcus aureus* in Melbourne hospitals in the late 1970s and early 1980s, *Antibiotic Guidelines* was compiled and distributed as a means to improve antibiotic usage. Antibiotic misuse was considered one of the reasons for the propagation of these resistant strains. The book was publicized in order to get its message across to practitioners. The *Guidelines* is now in its sixth edition and used throughout Australia.

by using vancomycin and initiating broad public health measures among hospital personnel and hospital services, the Melbourne hospitals were eventually able to contain the microorganism and its spread. But the problem remains prominent in hospitals there, where 20–40% of the *S. aureus* are still multiply resistant today. The Australians learned a lot from the experience. Public health measures did help control spread of these resistant bacteria. But everybody realized that antibiotic resistance could emerge as a devastating, nearly uncontrollable health problem. In this Melbourne epidemic, the "worst case" scenario was experienced.

What if this kind of event were to occur today? It is not out of the realm of possibility. Today, less than a decade later, vancomycin resistance has emerged in the microorganisms known as enterococci, which exchange other resistance genes with staphylococci. Moreover, vancomycin resistance is not confined to one kind of determinant. There are three different resistance determinants that can mediate vancomycin resistance, two of which are transferable. So far, resistance gene transfers from enterococci to staphylococci have not included vancomycin resistance. Still, the fact that such determinants now exist, that they are located on transferable plasmids and are appearing worldwide, is cause for serious concern. The relief from multiple resistance that vancomycin gave in the early 1980s may be short-lived, if these resistances spread into other bacteria, notably the staphylococci. No one can afford to be complacent. We must all take heed of these unusual but disastrous events and work toward preventing similar occurrences in the future.

As we mentioned earlier, another "close call" for antibiotics failure occurred in the early 1980s in Zaire, where multiresistant *Shigella dysenteriae*, which causes severe and often bloody diarrhea, claimed hundreds of lives. These infectious bacteria were resistant to all commonly used antibiotics. Only nalidixic acid was effective, and in many cases, it was administered too late. Moreover, within a year after nalidixic acid was introduced, strains resistant to this antimicrobial appeared and thwarted treatment. In this *Shigella* epidemic, however, it was the only drug available.

For some it was life-saving; for others it proved too late or altogether useless.

While these two examples may be regarded as isolated incidents, that is not the case. Other smaller outbreaks of hard-to-treat, resistant infections have surfaced in different parts of the world—in the general community, as well as in hospitals. Some of these we have discussed earlier—tuberculosis in New York, salmonellosis in Illinois. They offer a bleak picture for the future if such events start proliferating. An improvement in our understanding and acknowledgment of the resistance problem is needed to prevent such incidents from reaching calamitous proportions. Certain common features underlying the emergence and spread of antibiotic resistance merit comment.

LOW-LEVEL RESISTANCE PRECEDES HIGH-LEVEL RESISTANCE

Studies of certain respiratory and urinary tract pathogens alert us to an interesting biological phenomenon—low-level resistance precedes high-level resistance. At the International Congress of Infectious Diseases a few years ago, Dr. Fernando Baquero of the Hospital Ramon y Cajal in Madrid, showed that the first penicillin-resistant strains of meningococcus, gonococcus, and even pneumococcus that appeared were only slightly less susceptible (more resistant) than the susceptible strains. In most cases, these low-level mutants were not of concern because the resistance could be overwhelmed with a high dose of antibiotic. Following closely on the heels of these low-level resistant variants, however, were those with higher resistances. What had happened was that, with time, these or other strains had picked up genes having more powerful mechanisms of resistance to these antibiotics, namely those on plasmids and on transposons. Dr. Baquero proposed that we should pay more attention to these low-level resistant variants when they are seen in hospital or clinic bacteriology units because they usually herald the eventual appearance of the higher-level, resistant types that truly compromise treatment. A similar picture has emerged with quinolone resistance. Many more mutants with low-level resistance have emerged than those that resist therapeutic levels of the drugs. Unless you look carefully for these low-level resistant mutants, you will not identify them easily. In the case of quinolone resistance, low-level mutants do not pick up new resistant genes but show a greatly increased ability to emerge with mutations in their own chromosomes that confer a high level of resistance that thwarts treatment. Mutation directly to high-level resistance is not common in the parental bacterial strains. Thus, clinically relevant high-level quinolone resistant mutants appear to emerge in two mutational steps: the first gives low-level resistance, probably from a membrane impermeability to the drug, and the second provides high-level resistance via a change in the DNA gyrase—the enzyme target of the quinolones—making the cell resistant to the quinolones.

In most resistant bacteria, the level of antibiotic resistance expressed is far higher than what is actually needed to resist a therapeutic dose of antibiotics. The resistance determinants are providing an excess of resistance power. It is like taking a mallet to kill a fly. This finding suggests that the evolution of resistance determinants was probably not merely a response to accommodate the antibiotic levels that we use. Perhaps it was not even for the purpose of fighting antibiotics. These determinants may actually have another function in nature that eludes scientific investigators. In any case, they become more frequent when they are selected by the antibiotics to which they render their bacterial hosts resistant.

ONE ANTIBIOTIC CAN SELECT FOR RESISTANCE TO OTHERS

There is another feature of resistance that adds to the problem. Since most plasmids and even many transposons contain genes for resistance to different antibiotics, the use of any one of these antibiotics will select bacteria with resistance to all of them. This event will occur immediately if the multiresistant bacteria are already there. But, even if they are not initially evident, they can be recruited, as we discussed before, by chronic use of a single antibiotic. While initially, the drug selects bacteria resistant to itself, with time multiple resistance emerges from genes acquired elsewhere. And, as noted earlier, tetracycline or chloramphenicol can select *Escherichia coli* mutants without acquired resistant genes that are resistant via a chromosome mutation not only to the antibiotic doing the selection, but also to others *unrelated* to it. Of particular note, among the resistances so selected is low-level resistance to the quinolones. These mutants are at the first step on the path to high-level quinolone resistance, which we discussed before. If the use of one antibiotic can indirectly select mutants to others, even to the newest drugs, we can see that the resistance problem, in all its complexity, poses an immense challenge to the future.

DISCOVER NEW DRUGS AND NEW APPROACHES

To address and deal with the present resistance problems, investigators in drug research have immersed themselves in the task of discovering and developing new antibiotics that are not subject to known antibiotic resistance mechanisms. If a drug is totally new, resistance mechanisms may not yet have been selected. But such truly "new" antibiotics are becoming harder and harder to find. Researchers seeking new antibiotics among bacteria and fungi in soils often end up discovering the same kinds of antibiotics that have been found before, or subtle variations of them. If the drug does not differ greatly from prior antibiotics, it will be thwarted by resistance mechanisms already in existence.

The leaders of recent drug discovery programs are now casting their nets elsewhere to find new antibiotics. One potential source is in the new kinds of bacteria recovered from drilling miles beneath the earth's surface. Another innovative source is insects from which antibiotic-like substances have been discovered recently. Meanwhile, other investigators have identified antibacterial compounds in the skin of frogs. Scientists were led to these substances by observing that frogs did not become infected after surgery and placement back into water in which bacteria were prominent. Extracts of the skin provided the answer—antibiotic substances now called "magainins." Curiously, yet another group of new antibiotics was recently found in our own white cells, the neutrophils, which circulate in our blood. These substances have been called "defensins" since they act to defend the body against bacteria, viruses, and fungi.

These new types of "antibiotics," such as magainins and defensins, offer some optimism because they differ strikingly from those currently in use. For now, they are made only in small amounts. The goal is to produce these new antibiotic substances in large enough quantities to be used therapeutically against infection. Since they are made of protein, however, it is of some concern that they may be recognized by the body as foreign and removed by antibodies of the person's immune system. Moreover, as with other antibiotics, these new ones risk succumbing to the same ecological fate—the selection of mutants resistant to them. The likelihood and time frame for the appearance of such mutants will depend not only on the nature of the antibiotic itself, but also on how much and how often it is used. It is not surprising that the more a killing agent is used, the more likely it is to select a rare mutant that can resist it. Still, the finding of truly new agents is an important advance.

Other findings also support optimism. Some resistant bacterial strains may be able to accommodate one kind of resistance but not others. More specifically, resistance to some antibiotics may increase the bacterium's susceptibility to others. But which ones are they? Shouldn't we find out? Perhaps once bacteria become resistant to one drug, they become more sensitive to another. Evidence for this kind of phenomenon has come from studies of tetracycline resistance. Bacteria resistant to tetracycline by means of a membrane protein that pumps tetracycline out of the cell, are

more susceptible to aminoglycoside antibiotics, such as kanamycin and gentamicin. These kinds of antibiotics are used clinically with caution within very defined maximal levels because of
their inherent toxicity to the kidney. If less of these antibiotics
could be used, the side effects would be greatly reduced and their
efficacy would be improved. In a still more unexpected example,
salicylates, the ingredient in aspirin, can cause some bacteria to
increase resistance to certain antibiotics, but at the same time gain
sensitivity to others. We could profit from devoting some time to
looking at the consequences to the host bacterium of bearing
resistance to an antibiotic. While the resistance mechanism
may be helpful in the face of the antibiotic, it may be a detriment
to other functions of the bacteria. The resistance may reduce the
bacterium's ability to cause disease by causing changes in its cell
wall. For example, research scientists noted that some pneumococci that became more resistant to penicillin by cell wall
changes were less able to produce disease. A microorganism
called *Bordetella*, which causes the disease tularemia, has resistance and virulence genes intricately linked. Mutations in one or
more genes have the potential to create negative consequences on
others in this bacterium. Some of these negative effects may be
subtle, and are presently unknown. If discovered, they could be
used to an advantage. For instance, knowing that bacteria bearing
a resistance trait can no longer live at a particular temperature or
in a particular acid or basic environment could allow us to develop
alternative ways to destroy them. In other words, treatment can be
aimed directly at those bacteria bearing a particular resistance
determinant.

A different research approach has attempted to produce
drugs that will cure bacteria of their resistance elements. For
instance, certain chemicals inhibit the multiplication of plasmids.
If the plasmid is not duplicated, each new daughter cell will
theoretically be free of the plasmid and its linked resistances.
But this approach is up against a major stumbling block. While
many of these resistance determinants lie on extrachromosomal
DNA elements, such as plasmids, they also reside on chromo-

somes in the form of transposons. Therefore, the curing of a plasmid will never assure removal of the determinant. Since it lies on a transposon, it can be transferred onto another chromosome where it will remain stable. If we go after the chromosome, we are essentially doing what antibiotics do—killing the bacterial cell.

Natural selection has already complicated this approach. Genetic studies by Ron Skurray and his research team in Melbourne, Australia showed how resistance genes, formerly on plasmids, have moved onto chromosomes of resistant staphylococci. This movement to the chromosomes has had two major effects, one for the determinant and the other for the cell. When the resistance gene is on the chromosome, it is more stable. It is no longer susceptible to the vagaries of a plasmid that can be lost spontaneously by the cell. By moving onto the chromosome, the determinant and the cell no longer need the plasmid. The cell, in losing its resistance plasmids, can then accommodate other plasmids more easily—namely, those bearing new resistances. Thus, like a new book in a library, a new resistance gene first enters the cell and circulates freely on the plasmid. With time, it is put out of rapid circulation into the chromosome, the cell's "permanent noncirculating collection" (Figure 8.2).

There is, of course, the possibility of designing a compound that would specifically interfere with the replication of transposons. One way is to introduce genetic material that interrupts the duplication and/or spread of the transposon. If transposons could be eliminated, such treatments could selectively remove a multitude of resistance determinants from their natural reservoirs, whether they be on chromosomes or plasmids. Because the approach deals with transposons and not the entire bacterial cell, it would maintain the natural ecology of the normally harmless bacterial host strains, such as the skin and intestinal flora. It would not lead to a change in the normal flora. Instead of killing, it would act by selectively removing the "passenger" resistance genes. The approach would maintain this important normal skin and intestinal flora, which protect us from invasion by more harmful varieties. If cured of their transferable resistances, these bacteria

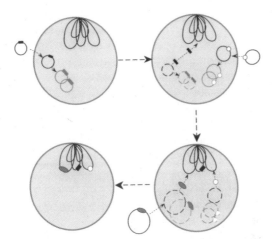

Figure 8.2. In *Staphylococcus aureus*, resistance genes enter on plasmids that multiply. Later in time, the genes find a place on the chromosome. This event allows other plasmids of similar types to enter with different resistance genes. This phenomenon has led to the recruitment of multiple genes for resistance in a single *S. aureus* strain (Bonnie Marshall, Tufts University School of Medicine).

would no longer pose the threat of transferring resistance to more harmful bacteria that might enter these areas.

RATIONAL DESIGN OF NEW DRUGS

Scientists and clinicians must stay ahead in this struggle with microbes by discovering both new antibiotics and uncovering novel ways to combat resistance. They must find a way to make the best use of the antibiotics now available, while seeking alternative approaches and new drugs. One approach has been to introduce chemical changes into members of the present array of antibiotics so that they are no longer modifiable by the enzymes associated with resistance. The historic example is methicillin, developed to resist penicillin-degrading enzymes.

A more recent example is the new family of quinolones that

are totally synthetic. They take their core structure from the first member of the quinolone group, nalidixic acid, the drug used in the *Shigella* epidemic in Zaire. As we mentioned, this synthetic group, discovered in the 1960s, lost favor because bacteria became spontaneously resistant to it at a frequency of about one in ten million. This is too high when hundreds of millions of bacteria could be involved. In contrast, the new quinolones do not select for resistance at anywhere near that frequency—more like one in 1 billion to one in 100 billion—a frequency much less apt to occur during therapy. Another seemingly protective feature of those quinolone resistant mutants that have emerged is that the resistance determinants are found on the chromosome. Here the resistance determinant has less chance of moving to other bacteria— not the case for those resistance genes that can be transferred on transposons or plasmids.

Another avenue for assaulting resistance is to design decoy molecules to fool the resistance mechanism. The enzyme "zeroes in" on something that looks like penicillin. It hooks onto it and busily tries to destroy the false target while penicillin sneaks in unscathed to kill the cell. The use of β-lactam chemicals, such as clavulanic acid or sulbactam, to compete for or block the β-lactamase enzymes that destroy penicillins has revitalized the efficacy of ampicillin, ticarcillin, and other broad spectrum penicillins. These penicillins suffer in the grasp of degradative enzymes in the resistant bacteria. Similar kinds of false substrates can be designed to attack other resistance mechanisms, such as those that involve other enzymes that modify and inactivate antibiotics, or other membrane proteins that actively export the antibiotic out of the cell.

NEW DRUGS MAY BE SUBJECT TO THE ACTIVITY OF OLD RESISTANCE DETERMINANTS

A setback to new discovery is the relatively recent observation that resistance to the newer drugs is appearing faster than ever expected. Within less than a decade, resistances have compromised use of the newer cephalosporins, penicillins, trimethoprim, and trimethoprim-sulfamethoxazole combinations, and the new aminoglycosides.

New drugs, introduced into the clinical arena, may run into a resistance "roadblock" within as short a period as two years. Why? Part of the answer relates to their heavy usage and the selection of resistance as with other drugs. Mass marketing takes place in order to sell enough of the new drug to make up for the large expense of developing it. A new drug becomes a "fad," something physicians (and their patients) want to use. Thus, large amounts of drug are presented to the bacterial ecosystem—just the right selective force for propagating the rare mutants bearing resistance mechanisms for that drug.

Another part of the problem is the lack of structural uniqueness in these new drugs. Generally, newly discovered drugs are tested and designed to be invulnerable to the known resistance determinants. If a new drug, however, is structurally related to an older one, the new antibiotic may eventually be inactivated by the same old resistance mechanisms. Under heavy use, the drug may select for rare mutant forms of these "old" resistance determinants— mutant proteins that can now inactivate the newer form of the antibiotic (Figure 8.3). This possibility was vividly brought home in the recent emergence of resistances to the newest penicillins and cephalosporins. In Germany, a plasmid encoding resistance to the new cephalosporins appeared in a clinical strain of *Klebsiella*, a potential cause of pneumonias and systemic infections. A genetic study showed that the gene for the enzyme that degraded the antibiotic was the same as one that destroyed the simpler, older cephalosporins. A couple of mutations in the gene for the enzyme had occurred which extended the structural forms of cephalosporins that the enzyme could destroy.

The best reconstruction of events leading to this new determinant would be that random mutations occurred during the many duplications of the old resistance gene. In most cases these mutations would be inconsequential and would be diluted out by all the normal genes. One of these mutations, however, allowed the

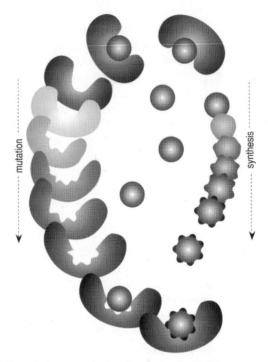

Figure 8.3. Bacteria have acquired resistance genes for β-lactamases which are able to break down newer forms of penicillins and cephalosporins. β-Lactamases with an increased spectrum of activity result from small mutations in a previous β-lactamase gene with a narrower spectrum of activity. The new protein now accommodates and destroys the newer β-lactam antibiotics (Bonnie Marshall, Tufts University School of Medicine).

bacteria to survive in the presence of the new cephalosporin antibiotic. These bacteria propagated under the antibiotic selection. Once the new gene became a significant part of the environmental pool of resistance, it could be transferred to other bacteria and the persistence of the new resistance determinant would be assured.

Another example comes from a number of outbreaks in different countries of resistant intestinal bacteria capable of destroying the newer generation of penicillins. Again, genetic analysis showed these genes to be mutations of the very common TEM-1 β-lactamase gene—the gene that specifies an enzyme that breaks the β-lactam ring of penicillins and so inactivates the antibiotic. Natural mutations, at rates of one in a million to one in 100 million, had led to a form of the enzyme that could detoxify all of these new drugs. Like the cephalosporin-degrading enzymes, these "new" penicillin-destructive enzymes have become increasingly evident.

These β-lactamase changes are examples of how evolution (in this case that of a single gene) combined with strong antibiotic selection, can forge new resistances from old resistance determinants. Today, more than two dozen different TEM-1-like β-lactamases have emerged. Members of this new family of resistance enzymes can destroy the old penicillins as well as any of the new penicillin derivatives currently on the market. This will probably extend to others making their way into clinical practice. Thus, they threaten the therapeutic use and efficacy of these newer antibiotics.

FROM DISCOVERY TO APPLICATION IS TIME-CONSUMING AND EXPENSIVE

The optimists believe that the vista for drug discoveries is limitless and that we will continue to find new ones to deal with resistance problems. The pessimists say "Let's be practical. The money needed to find these new drugs and the time required to put them into use is very long and very costly." With each new drug there is a chance of high toxicity. In fact, the vast majority of drugs never reach clinical use because of their toxic side effects when ingested or injected. The discovery and development process is a lengthy one, which could prevent the entry of new drugs into the market fast enough to keep up with the mounting problem of resistance. It usually takes over ten years for a new drug to leave the development stage and move into clinical practice. Only about 4–5% of new medicines ever make it into use. To get final approval from the Food and Drug Administration and similar agencies worldwide, companies must perform scores of time-consuming studies and complete reams of paperwork. Millions of dollars must be spent for all the studies needed before the drug actually reaches the marketplace. Besides demonstrating that the new antibiotic can kill certain bacteria, these drugs must be tested in animals to show that they cause no harm; only then are they tested in humans, both for efficacy and toxicity. If it can pass the human "trials," the new drug finally makes it into the marketplace. Given these enormous constraints, even if one were to design an ideal drug today to deal with current antibiotic resistance problems, the drug would not be available for another decade. Even then there is no guarantee it would still be effective.

One patient related that he asked his physician, "Won't these drugs become useless if we use them too much?" His doctor replied, "There is no need to worry. We have so many antibiotics available and new ones are being discovered all the time." While this may have been true during the heyday of antibiotic discovery, it is certainly not true now when new antibiotics are coming into the clinical arena so slowly.

A WORLD WITH NO ANTIBIOTIC CONTROLS

It is somewhat fanciful to wonder, but perhaps worth considering, what would happen if there were no controls on antibiotic use and all people were freely able to use antibiotics at their own whims. Susceptible strains would be totally eliminated and resistant ones would dominate. Would the resistant bacteria survive? It appears that they would. There is very little evidence to suggest that resistant bacteria are less able to compete in an ecosystem than their susceptible siblings. In this imaginary situation, the levels of resistant bacteria would be so high that use of any antibiotic would not be effective, given the predominance of microorganisms with resistance.

The place where the antibiotic resistant strain has emerged—a hospital, community, or country—would be a source of protection from spread, *if* this location could be quarantined. Unfortunately, in most cases, this would be difficult to achieve. Imagine that a country, let's say in Southeast Asia, is struggling with high numbers of multiple antibiotic-resistant disease-causing bacteria that in most people, cannot be eliminated by any antibiotic. Some people in the environment could become inadvertent "carriers" of these bacteria, since not all people would get disease from them. This situation would lead to the movement of these strains into new communities, and potentially, anywhere else in the world. Such is the case of the typhoid fever bacillus resistant to ampicillin, the best antibiotic then used to treat this disease, which appeared in patients in Los Angeles in the mid-1970s. It was later traced to Mexico, where these patients had been visiting. As noted earlier, public health officials have been able to identify brothels in Southeast Asia as the initial source of penicillin-resistant bacteria causing gonorrhea, which are now found in virtually every country of the world.

If we imagined an earth totally bathed in antibiotics, the only bacteria surviving would be those resistant to these drugs. The end result would be a reestablished microbial world carrying on its usual activity, except that all members of this microbial population, both helpful and harmful, would be untouched by the very antibiotics to which their less fortunate ancestors had succumbed. For this new "breed" of bacteria, antibiotics would be ineffective, merely a part of their environment. Antibiotics would fit into the category of environmental toxins with which bacteria would be interacting without harm during everyday activity. A new, stable evolutionary change would be established with bacteria remaining untouched by antibiotics. In fact, this is exactly how *Escherichia coli* already deal with many of the toxic elements in our gastrointestinal tract—the *E. coli* outer wall coat keeps out toxic chemicals, such as bile salts.

Even today, certain bacteria have emerged with resistance to one or more antibiotics as a common characteristic. More than 90% of the species of *Proteus mirabilis* are now tetracycline resistant. In an analogous situation, more than 90% of *Staphylococcus aureus* resist penicillin, making penicillin ineffective against the vast majority of this species. Given what we are seeing already, it is not difficult to envision a total microbial change in favor of resistant forms. Under these circumstances, unless humans developed a solid immunity to bacteria, we would face a dreaded time when our ability to treat infections would be doomed to failure. The world might seem like a replay of the uncontrollable plagues of the Dark Ages.

To some extent, this scenario has already come to pass in developing countries among the indigent populations. In these areas, death is a preponderant part of life. Poor sanitation leads to spread of infectious agents while antibiotic misuse propagates resistant strains. To make matters worse, these are the very countries where money is so scarce that the government cannot afford to buy the currently useful but expensive antibiotics. People are dying from diseases that were previously treatable. Can a similar situation ever threaten the affluent, developed world?

Under the present circumstances, we can extend our imagination to a situation where multiresistant microorganisms would become so dominant and of such concern that individuals would have to be checked and decontaminated microbiologically before they passed between countries. Years ago I considered such a scene to be ridiculous and totally farfetched. Today, at a time when China and the United States are asking that applicants for certain visas announce whether or not they have been infected by the AIDS virus, and other countries may demand that visitors show evidence of a recent AIDS antibody test, such ideas join the realm of possibility.

Imagine you are returning from a country where it is known that infectious agents with multiple resistances dwell. An example could be a *Staphylococcus aureus*, which is resistant to all available antibiotics, including vancomycin (the one drug left to treat this common hospital scourge). You might be asked to enter an isolation room, take a shower or be otherwise sanitized before you are finally released (Figure 8.4). Many would look back fondly on the good days long gone when all you had to do was wait in line to fill out an immigration card and get your passport stamped. Trips would be lengthened not only by security checks at departure, but by a new kind of security check upon arrival.

A paradigm of this situation does exist in Perth, Australia. In order to safeguard their hospitals from multiply resistant *Staphylococcus aureus*, medical personnel place all new patients entering any hospital in Perth into an isolation area first. There the patient

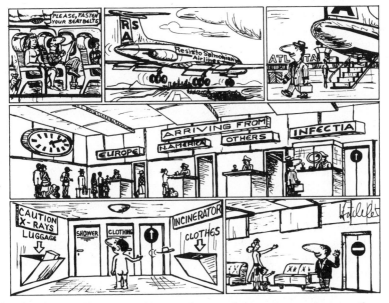

Figure 8.4. Will we ever reach a time when entering a country requires more than passport control? (Herbert Hächler, University of Zurich, Zurich, Switzerland).

is tested for the presence of the methicillin-resistant *Staphylococcus aureus* (MRSA). Those new patients who are not colonized by MRSA can go on to the normal hospital wards. If a MRSA microorganism is found on a patient, however, this person is placed in a ward with other patients colonized with this potentially dangerous and easily spread microorganism. Various means are used to eradicate the microorganism. Nonetheless, if the patient has an indwelling catheter or other foreign object in place, no treatment can eliminate all of the microorganisms that find hiding places in and on these objects. In such instances, the patient must stay in these designated MRSA areas throughout the hospitalization.

By this single measure of isolating patients with MRSA, the hospitals in Perth have kept MRSA under control and the frequency of these strains is now among the lowest in the world. This draconian measure to control the early spread of bacteria has worked, but not without psychological consequences for the patients involved. Still, the success of this practice has led to its being suggested as a means to control the early spread of resistant bacteria. It is certainly one proven avenue for controlling the entry of resistant strains into a new area, such as other hospital wards. How to effectively prevent *spread* from a larger affected area, such as whole regions or countries, to other areas is much harder to envision.

HOW DO WE PROTECT THE FUTURE FROM RESISTANCE?

We, in all segments of society, must try to adhere to certain principles to safeguard our future and those of future generations. Let us outline certain goals that will help us achieve a brighter outcome.

1. Consumers should use antibiotics only when needed, at the correct dosage, and for the prescribed time period.

2. Medical associations and schools should provide continued and updated education on current antibiotic uses to prescribers and users. This can be done by including these subjects for discussion and presentation at medical meetings and as up-to-date lectures to medical, dental, veterinary, and agricultural students.

3. Research scientists and drug manufacturers should continue to acquire insights into the mechanisms of resistance and the factors associated with their spread. With this information, investigators can begin to design ways to circumvent these resistances and to prevent their spread. One approach is to design antibiotic substrates that block, trick, and confound the resistance mechanisms.

4. Pharmaceutical companies should be encouraged, even by tax and patent advantages, to discover new antibiotics for which resistance mechanisms have not yet emerged.

5. Medical personnel should develop alternatives to antibiotics to treat infectious diseases. Vaccines against common bacterial diseases and improved public health measures worldwide will do much to decrease reliance on, and overuse of, antibiotics.

6. Public health authorities should improve public sanitation, especially water quality, in developing areas of the world where the spread of infectious diseases is high and where antibiotics are clearly needed.

7. Surveillance of clinical isolates should be instituted or performed on a regular basis. This helps epidemiologists identify areas of endemic resistance and aids doctors in the selection of appropriate antibiotics. Together they can limit spread to nonendemic areas.

The phenomenon of antibiotic resistance, including the genetics, resistance mechanisms, and their rampant spread, must be fully understood in order to protect the world population from what could become a plague of resistance. Scientists are fervently taking steps to procure this knowledge. The obstacles, however, still challenge the most determined scientists.

Part of the responsibility for appropriate antibiotic use certainly rests on all of us. The consequences of misuse affect ourselves, our families, and our communities. The truly unsettling feature of misuse is the selection of resistant bacterial strains. They will inflict harm not only on the present-day population but also on generations to follow and potentially, on a worldwide basis. We must curtail the creation of new resistant strains that, once selected, join the microbial population at large. Moreover, we must contain them once they are recognized. Above all, we must set our goals to limit practices that select and propagate antibiotic resistance.

Chapter 9

THE INDIVIDUAL AND ANTIBIOTIC RESISTANCE

The problem with medicating yourself is that you don't know what you're doing.

Anonymous

An antibiotic-resistant infection is no longer an unexpected or curious phenomenon for community physicians to observe in their patients. People of all ages and with various illnesses are becoming aware that antibiotics are no longer all-powerful. More and more parents of young children suffering from ear infections are finding that the prior successes of the penicillin drugs in treating this illness may not be repeated. They must now rely on other more costly drugs to which they may have a toxic reaction.

Major new advances in curing cancer have been thwarted and undermined by the emergence of bacterial infections that fail to respond to old and new antibiotics alike. Thus, although the cancer may have been controlled or even cured, some 25–30% of patients may die from infectious agents, of which half may be caused by bacteria resistant to current antibiotic therapy.

Patients admitted to the hospital for organ transplants may find their course of treatment compromised by unrelenting infections that would have responded previously to effective and safe antibiotics. A person taking an antibiotic for one infection may contract another infection, this time a resistant one, through contamination of food products or through "pick up" from other people or animals in the environment. In sum, resistant forms of bacteria are all around us. We must learn to cope with them and to develop ways of reducing their numbers.

Because of the power by which antibiotics "select for" resistant bacteria, every person taking an antibiotic potentially contributes a bit to the environmental pool of resistant bacteria. Some do so more than others. We are, therefore, not innocent victims of the antibiotic resistance phenomenon. Moreover, each person taking an antibiotic *inappropriately* plays a larger role in the resistance problem since this is an *unnecessary* selection of antibiotic resistance. From some public health estimates, this inappropriate use may be as much as half the number of times antibiotics are currently taken.

Many people believe that hospitals are havens for resistant infections. They are not necessarily wrong; however, a common source of resistant hospital strains are the newly admitted patients themselves. More specifically, they or their bacterial flora are the barometers of antibiotic use in the community and, therefore, reflect the frequency of resistance there.

It may be disturbing to learn that any use of an antibiotic, whether appropriate or not, will do its own share of selecting resistant forms of bacteria. It would be absurd to jump from this fact to a judgment that antibiotics should, therefore, not be used. We must accept some resistance as a natural consequence of use. But "some" level of resistance is potentially controllable. It need not be widespread, nor does it have to be multiple, that is, to more than one antibiotic. Our principal goal is to improve antibiotic use so as to maintain efficacy at the same time that we whittle away at resistance. Appropriate use of antibiotics can eliminate the causative infectious bacteria without major consequences to the environment. Advances in knowledge are evolving to help us. For one thing, as we have discussed before, short-term use has fewer ecologic effects, in terms of selecting multiresistant bacteria, than does chronic use for weeks at a time. In the right setting, for certain urinary tract infections, a single day's treatment is enough to cure the infection. In this instance, the antibiotic chosen needs to be one that is heavily concentrated in the urine. Its effectiveness is assured by drinking lots of fluids and repeated voiding of the bacteria in the urine. The major effect of the antibiotic is to inhibit the bacterium's ability to cling to the wall of the bladder.

On the other hand, too short a treatment, such as for pneumonia or a bone infection, would allow infectious bacteria to survive and reinfect, with potentially decreased susceptibility to the antibiotic treatment. For example, incomplete treatment is one of the presumed causes of multidrug-resistant tuberculosis facing the world today. Therefore, an understanding of the dynamics of antibiotic activity and antibiotic selection of resistance can help lead us to use these valuable drugs successfully and safely, yet prudently.

The world population has used antibiotics for over 40 years. The enthusiasm following the success of the sulfonamides in the 1930s was heightened by the discovery of penicillin's effectiveness in the 1940s. These events are within the current memory of people living now. The idea that there is such an entity as a "miracle drug" that will cure all ailments remains with us, even among prescribers. The editors of the French medical journal, *La Revue Prescrire*, which aims to improve standards of medical prescription in France, illustrated this fact vividly in an experiment a few years ago. In an example of advertising power and reader gullibility, the journal, on April Fool's Day, advertised a pill *Panaceum* that, with one dosage, would control mental illness for a year. Unexpectedly, within days of its publication, pharmacies in France were bombarded with inquiries and orders from willing believers who were all too ready to prescribe, as well as to swallow, such a "magic" pill. Gilles Bardelay, the editor of *Prescrire*, had to go on public television to explain the joke—one he thought would have been perfectly obvious (Figure 9.1).

INDIVIDUAL ACCESSIBILITY AND USE OF ANTIBIOTICS

To many individuals, the word antibiotic, not just penicillin, still means a drug that will cure diseases of all kinds. They do not distinguish between bacterial or other causes of the illness. This belief is, of course, as we have mentioned repeatedly, completely false. For instance, the average person will seek an antibiotic for relief of flu symptoms, caused by a virus. As we have noted, if an antibiotic is obtainable without prescription, as in many countries in Central and South America and in Asia, the patient can buy it directly over the counter at the local pharmacy.

In most industrialized countries such as the United States, antibiotics for human consumption are available only by prescrip-

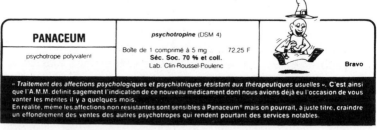

Figure 9.1. The April 1984 issue of the French medical journal, *La Revue Prescrire*, came out on April Fool's Day. It advertised a new psychotropic drug called *Panaceum* that could control mental illness for a year. While it was intended as a joke, the overwhelming response from physicians and pharmacies wanting to know where and how to get this drug required the editor of the magazine to make a public disclaimer (*La Revue Prescrire*, Paris, France).[1]

tion. This practice is dictated by law because this group of drugs can have certain toxic side effects, including allergies, for which care by a physician is necessary. It is even possible to die from some of these reactions. Some of the drugs can be given only intravenously and, therefore, the patient needs expert medical facilities, usually a hospital. Finally, control over prescription drugs may have been envisioned to avoid indiscriminate use and subsequent selection of resistant forms of bacteria. The effectiveness of this safeguard is now in question.

We may ask how much of the antibiotics used in the United States come through physicians' prescriptions and how much otherwise. Perhaps not surprisingly, there is a major proportion of the latter. For example, one investigation into the problem of antibiotic-resistant gonorrhea in a Baltimore venereal disease clinic found that 10% of patients had already taken antibiotics during the two weeks before they attended the clinic. Seventy percent of these patients took the antibiotics because they suspected they "might" have a venereal disease; the other 30% took antibiotics for other reasons. When tested, only 5 of the 61 patients who took antibiotics actually harbored the gonococcus. Of these, all but one had an antibiotic-resistant infection, as compared with only 31% of the 121 patients who had not taken an antibiotic. More interesting, perhaps, was the finding that half the patients previously on an antibiotic had procured it through channels *other* than a health care provider. We cannot say whether the prior antibiotic use cured the majority of ingestors without detectable gonococcus or whether they never had infections. It is noteworthy, however, that so many were able to get the drugs without prescription—and in the United States at that. More importantly, the authors of this study concluded that, "the combined influences of relatively frequent self-administration of antibiotics . . . may have helped to accelerate the pace at which antibiotic-resistant *Neisseria gonorrhoeae* emerged in Baltimore."[2]

If antibiotics are "prescribed-only" drugs, how do individuals gain access to them? There are many ways, not the least of which is storing and using leftover drugs. When I ask people what they do with medicines they do not take, the vast majority respond that they keep them for later use. They do not find the question or the answer embarrassing, only curious. In any number of homes, should you open the mirrored bathroom cabinets, you'll find bottles of unused drug tablets and liquids. This is not uncommon. One family showed me some tetracycline that was outdated. There is not any guarantee of its effectiveness, let alone its safety. And in the case of tetracycline, as it ages, it converts to a chemical which could cause toxic liver damage if taken.

People everywhere rely on antibiotics for different reasons— appropriately and inappropriately. Current practices do not always follow valid and prudent use, as the following examples will illustrate.

One woman came to the dermatology clinic at a local university-based hospital wanting treatment for a minor acne problem developing on her face. The resident physician informed her that the skin problem could be controlled by careful washing, proper skin care, and diet. There was no need for special medication. The patient became indignant and angrily demanded a prescription for tetracycline, a drug she knew by name because she had gotten it so many times before. The resident tried to explain to her why he advised against taking tetracycline for her minor skin problem. There was the risk of side effects, such as increased sensitivity to sunlight and a vaginal yeast infection. "But I want tetracycline," she exclaimed, pounding her fist on the clinic examining bed. The resident did not yield. Exasperated, the patient began screaming. "I want TETRACYCLINE . . . TETRACYCLINE!" which continued relentlessly despite attempts to calm her. Her shouts became even louder as the physician and nurse, embarrassed, hurriedly escorted her out (Figure 9.2).

Clearly, this is an example of the extreme to which a patient might go in order to obtain treatment. This patient's faith in tetracycline, coupled with her strong desire to clear up a flaw in her physical appearance, temporary as it was, led her to try to intimidate the physician into prescribing the medication. Under

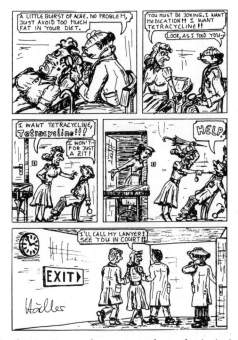

Figure 9.2.   Antibiotic misuse—the consumer demands. An insistent patient can be a problem to the physician and to the clinical establishment (Herbert Hächler, University of Zurich, Zurich, Switzerland).

different circumstances, in another setting, such an action might have been successful.

*   *   *   *   *

A Washington businessman on his second plane trip to New York in three days felt a scratchiness in his throat. Without looking up from his work, he took a penicillin tablet out of the sidepocket of his briefcase and swallowed it with his complimentary coffee. He was certain that this precaution would prevent his coming down with a full-fledged cold.

One pill would have no effect on an incipient throat infection, even if it were bacterial. In this case, it was probably a viral cold. Add to that his attitude, and that of the public in general, that such use is harmless. There is no concern for the side effects of such medications, or worry about using drugs that are out-dated, or of the selection of new resistant, infectious agents. The problem is that, in most cases, no harm *is* evident and so the practice continues. Multiply this one instance by all those individuals worldwide who keep antibiotics on hand and take them at the first symptom without physician advice and the magnitude of this indiscriminate use should become obvious.

*   *   *   *   *

A local real estate broker boasted that his mother has never had a problem getting any antibiotic she wants. "She first shops around until she finds a doctor who will write prescriptions for her."

A physician related a story relevant to this one. While he was looking after the patients of another physician who was on vacation, he was repeatedly asked by the patients to prescribe antibiotics for flu symptoms. When this covering physician refused because he did not think them necessary, the patients became upset. They complained to their own doctor when he returned. The covering physician was dismissed.

I recently asked a community physician about his experiences with antibiotic use on his own patients. "Patients ask for them by name," he replied. "It's tough not to give in to this pressure. Sometimes I do, sometimes I do not. It depends on how I feel about the situation and how I feel that day."

As these examples illustrate, physicians complain that they have difficulty dealing with the demands of patients who persist in their beliefs that they need antibiotics. As noted earlier, sometimes the physician rationalizes that maybe there is a bacterial infection as well as the cold virus. And, if he gives in, he will prescribe a relatively "safe" antibiotic, like penicillin or tetracycline. While the drug, in general, may be relatively harmless to that patient, it will cause major changes in the bacterial flora associated with the patient and, indirectly, that of the environment. There is also the potential of side effects, such as diarrhea, rashes, and headaches that certain individuals get with antibiotics. More general side effects, like nausea or stomach cramps, may also occur.

Whom do we blame, the physician or the patient, when an antibiotic is obtained for a common cold? People welcome the report from the automobile mechanic that all their car needed was an adjustment, a new spark plug, but not a total motor overhaul. We do not argue about paying for his time and expertise. Why then should patients be disappointed when the doctor says that their viral diseases need only aspirin, fluids, and rest? There is a certain irony in this practice, since in "playing doctor," these people make decisions that potentially endanger their health and possibly their lives.

*   *   *   *   *

A mother of ten children told me how she keeps her family healthy. "I keep a stock of penicillin suspensions and tablets in case of earaches and sore throats." "Do you ever consult your physician?" I asked. "Only if the child doesn't get better in a couple days," she replied.

It was a revelation to her to hear that penicillin and other miracle drugs were not always miraculous. There was a great chance of missing the correct cause of the infection. It might not even be bacterial. If it were, use of the antibiotic could preclude identifying the true cause of the ailment. One could not determine if the treatment was, at best, correct, or, at worst, a complication to curing it. The selection of resistant forms of bacteria in the household was not, of course, considered. She did not know that self-medication can be harmful and is often useless, certainly if an inadequate dosage is taken. And worse, it could help propagate a small amount of true disease agents into numbers large enough to cause infection.

*   *   *   *   *

A young mother in a Caribbean country witnessed her eight-year-old son being scratched by their cat. Although he was not upset, she became concerned about possible infection. She quickly loaded him into the car and headed to the doctor's office. There were fifteen people waiting ahead of her. "I wasn't going to wait." She told me. "He needed an antibiotic." So she went to a nearby pharmacy and obtained one. "Which one?" I asked. "I don't remember—one that the pharmacy had."

While we can understand the concern of the parent, we also see that she was taking her son's health into her own hands. What if the child had a reaction to the antibiotic? Perhaps she had chosen an antibiotic not to be used for children. Was an antibiotic really necessary? What about the possibility of a good scrubbing with soap, and a booster shot for tetanus?

CHANGING PATTERNS OF ANTIBIOTIC USE

The use of penicillins, namely ampicillin and amoxycillin, has risen in recent years in the United States.[3] This increase has occurred predominantly in the pediatric age group. The explanation for the increase is linked to the greater numbers of children attending day care centers, now that both parents typically work outside the home. In contrast to the times when children stayed at home or in smaller groups, the close child-to-child contact in these centers propagates the spread of common childhood diseases at earlier ages. This situation, antibiotic experts claim, has led to increased antibiotic usage. No one can be certain whether these illnesses are viral or bacterial, but antibiotics will be used often in any case. Thus, overall total annual antibiotic consumption goes up because it starts earlier and persists throughout the early years of school. This societal change puts additional pressure on the problem of selection of resistant bacteria. We do not criticize this change, but want only to increase awareness of its potential effect on the frequency of resistant infectious disease agents.

One research group in Texas compared the frequency of anti-biotic resistance among children in day care centers with that of children staying at home.[4] The investigators made a remarkable, but perhaps not totally unexpected finding. The level of resistant bacteria in the intestinal flora of the children in day care centers was at least twofold higher than that of children spending their days at home. Of particular interest, this higher level of resistance extended to relatively new antibiotics.

ANTIBIOTICS AND THE INDIVIDUAL'S BACTERIAL FLORA

The infectious virulence of a bacterium is not changed by its being resistant. The only thing that changes is the bacterium's ability to take hold in the body if an antibiotic to which it is resistant has been used. Nondisease-causing bacteria are essential parts of the body's natural "armor" against invading infectious bacteria (Figure 9.3). Once these are killed or diminished, resistant disease-causing bacteria can find a niche and multiply. Once they reach critical numbers, they can cause illness and, if resistant, will be harder to treat.

Our "protective" flora changes during the course of our activities and movements into new environments. We are constantly picking up and shedding bacteria. But these changes are of no consequence to our lives. If, during antibiotic therapy, we were to place ourselves within a germfree environment, bacterial exchanges with the outside would cease—we would be dealing only with our own bacterial flora. We could kill off all the susceptible microorganisms that we had and cause an increase only in the small numbers of resistant bacteria that were already there at the time the antibiotic was started. Once these resistant bacteria multiplied, reversion to a flora of susceptible bacteria would not be possible, since none could enter the germ-free environment. We could treat the resistant bacteria, if needed, with an appropriate

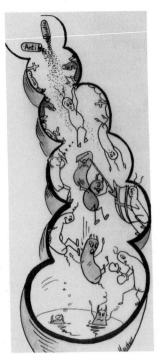

Figure 9.3. The bacteria lining the skin and intestinal tract form a protective "armor" against invasion by pathogens and other foreign bacteria. If, during antibiotic therapy, this protective coat is killed, resistant "invaders" have room to colonize and potentially cause disease problems (Bonnie Marshall, Tufts University School of Medicine).

antibiotic to which they were susceptible; however, we could do so without concern that other, resistant pathogenic bacteria would enter from the outside.

Obviously, the above scenario is, by and large, impractical; however, it is the reasoning now being applied in the treatment of cancer patients. When their bodies have become unable to cope with bacteria, they are placed in environments where entry of new bacteria is limited. These people are given diets of "cooked foods only," since these foods will be essentially free of bacteria. Living plants and flowers are removed from the rooms because bacteria which can potentially infect the patients may be present in them.

By this means, we curtail the entry of infectious agents and we monitor the kinds of bacteria already there. Thus, we know what kinds of bacteria will potentially cause an infection or a new fever and have the appropriate antibiotics on hand to treat them, if needed.

For an otherwise healthy individual, taking prescribed antibiotics in the home and community is not hazardous. Rigorous precautions against bacterial pick-up, as used in very sick people, are not needed. The natural defenses are intact and the chance of meeting up with a dangerously large number of resistant disease-causing bacteria is small. Moreover, once the antibiotic course is finished, susceptible strains will eventually return.

The level of susceptibility of the returning flora after antibiotic ingestion will, as we have mentioned, depend on the source of that flora, be it the immediate environment or foods that we eat. One study in France showed that when people who had relatively high numbers of resistant bacteria in their intestinal flora ate diets of only sterilized foods, their intestinal flora became more sensitive.[5] These findings suggest that the resistant flora we have may come from the food we eat, or that selective substances (antibiotics?) are in the food that help propagate resistant bacteria.

POTENTIAL INDIVIDUAL CONSEQUENCES OF ANTIBIOTIC USE

Probably the most significant unwanted consequence to the individual taking an antibiotic is the side effects that are inherent in all drugs. The chance of a side effect can be as high as 50%, depending on the drug. Many of these side effects, however, are so mild that we accept them in exchange for benefits we receive from the antibiotic. When taking an antibiotic, most people can deal with a little abdominal discomfort—nausea, cramps—especially when it subsides after several doses of the drug. The skin rash from penicillins may cause us to stop taking the drug but is not inherently serious. Other side effects, however, can be quite severe and unexpected, such as the life-threatening allergic reaction to penicillin, which is rare but carries a 30% death rate with it.

Prolonged use of some drugs can lead to toxicity in critical internal organs. Gentamicin, an excellent antibiotic for treating systemic bacterial infections, can cause damage to the kidneys. Streptomycin, used previously for many infections of the intestine, kidney, and lung, and now used primarily, if not exclusively, for tuberculosis, can lead to hearing defects. In a report from China, one physician attributed a large percentage of hearing defects in children to the overuse of streptomycin and other drugs from the same antibiotic class.[6]

Another side effect of antibiotic usage is the overgrowth of one's natural bacterial flora by other bacteria, including ones that produce toxins. Diarrhea caused by overgrowth of *Clostridium difficile* in the intestine follows treatment with broad-spectrum antibiotics to which this microorganism is resistant. The patient, already sick with one disease, now begins to suffer from painful and sometimes life-threatening diarrhea. Fortunately, we still have another antibiotic available to treat this problem, which is, ironically, the consequence of other antibiotic use.

Often, after prolonged use of broad-spectrum antibiotics, such as tetracycline, a secondary infection with yeast may appear. This is what produces the itching and pain in the vaginal area experienced by women being treated with tetracyclines or penicillins for a variety of ailments.

An unexpected consequence stemming from antibiotic use was exemplified in the *Salmonella* outbreaks in the United States that we discussed earlier (Chapter 6). Those people who happened to be on antibiotics when they consumed either contaminated meat or milk came down with severe diarrhea caused by an antibiotic-resistant *Salmonella*. Under the selective environment of the antibiotic, the resistant *Salmonella* reached sufficient numbers to cause gastroenteritis and, in some cases, blood infections resulting in death. Most people not taking an antibiotic, who had ingested the very same contaminated products, remained healthy and unaffected.

There are precautions that a healthy person can take to prevent this indirect consequence of antibiotic ingestion, that is, the "pick up" and propagation of these resistant bacteria. For instance, one can wash meats and cook them well before eating them. Uncooked fruits and vegetables can be prepared on different kitchen surfaces than those on which raw meats and fish have been processed. Because cooking will kill the bacteria, it is the uncooked foods that serve as a bacterial cocktail. Even minor contamination of these uncooked foods with small numbers of resistant bacteria from meat or fish could allow enough viable microorganisms to be ingested and enter the body. Concurrent use of an antibiotic would help them to propagate and potentially cause disease.

INDIVIDUAL EFFORTS AGAINST ANTIBIOTIC RESISTANCE

We are at a point in medical history where people expect a "pill for every ill." Some of the reasons for this attitude we have already discussed. Antibiotics do not help unless bacteria are involved in the problem. It is anti*bodies* made by our bodies, not anti*biotics* made by molds and soil bacteria, that protect and control viral infections and also serve in protecting us against repeated bacterial invasion.

Faced with this situation and the knowledge of how resistant bacteria are propagated and spread, each individual can help curtail this mounting world health problem. First of all and most directly, the individual must understand what an antibiotic can and cannot do. Antibiotics are treatment moieties for bacterial infections, that is, infections caused by microscopic single-cell microorganisms that cause disease when they get inside the body. These microorganisms disrupt normal physiological processes and can eventually lead to death. Antibiotics are superbly unique in being able to kill the bacteria while producing relatively little harm to the body of the ingestor, whether an animal, human, or plant.

An individual should know when, why, and for how long the prescribed antibiotic should be taken. He or she should ask these questions of the physician and then follow the directions for use. If the antibiotic is given to treat a bacterial infection, it needs to be taken for the entire course of therapy and not simply until the symptoms disappear. Resistant forms of the causative bacteria can emerge and increase in number if the drug is stopped before a treatment course is completed. Once these resistant forms are numerous, subsequent treatment with that antibiotic fails.

The existence of antibiotic resistance is hardly cause for total despair. Most antibiotics, even the older ones, can and do still have some effective uses today. They could have greater impact if the resistant strains were more outnumbered by the susceptible ones. The fear of resistance precludes the use of an antibiotic until the physician knows the infecting microorganisms are not resistant. This is a far cry from 20 years ago when just knowing what kind of microorganism caused the disease was enough to choose the appropriate antibiotic. Pharmaceutical companies, at least those that have remained in the antiinfective field, are still working hard toward discovering and developing new antibiotics. To a large extent, new antibiotics are being sought to circumvent resistance. Others are being derived to deal directly with the resistance mechanisms themselves. The ideal goal, from this point on, is for these new drugs to be used wisely and appropriately so as to limit the rate of selection and appearance of resistance.

Traditionally, antibiotic regimens last 5–10 days. New studies show how we can shorten the time that antibiotics must be taken in order to cure certain illnesses. As we have noted, many patients with uncomplicated urinary tract infections can be cured with only one day of oral antibiotic treatment. So, in this common community infection, short treatment works. Maybe there can be more examples like this, especially when given the appropriate antibiotic. This direction toward shorter courses would limit the environmental presence and selective effect these drugs would have on the emergence of multiresistant bacteria. New tests will allow physicians to diagnose infectious agents early enough to know exactly which antibiotic to use and for how long. Vaccine development can lead to prevention of diseases for which antibiotics are now needed.

Antibiotics remain effective agents in curing bacterial diseases. They have revolutionized medical therapy and are a major stalwart against infectious agents. But we must use them prudently and appropriately to curtail the rate of emergence of resistance to new drugs and prevent spread of resistance among totally unrelated bacteria. Once the antibiotics are in the hands of the patients, the patients assume the responsibility for themselves and their families. They must follow the directions for use. The consequences of antibiotic misuse come back to haunt the misuser as well as a multitude of innocent bystanders in the community, most notably other family members.

We have seen how individuals and communities have been ravaged by the consequences of irresponsible abuse of antibiotics. People worldwide are finally beginning to understand this problem and to deal with it. Producers, prescribers, and consumers are all taking a greater part in curtailing antibiotic abuse. By using these drugs effectively, each one of us protects the world population from the continued emergence and spread of resistance determinants. We must take responsibility for using antibiotics properly, since this will protect the future health of ourselves, our families, and our whole society.

Chapter 10

ANTIBIOTIC RESISTANCE

A Societal Issue at Local, National, and International Levels

Antibiotic resistance is not constrained by local or even national borders. It confronts all individuals and populations around the world. The answer to the problem must come from all societal groups. Misuse and overuse of antibiotics—whether in homes, hospitals, communities, in animal populations, or in agriculture— can provide the additional environmental force to select for and maintain resistant strains of bacteria (Figure 10.1). The killing effect of antibiotics is so strong that only the resistant bacteria will survive. When it is the consequence of treatment, we can accept it, and it is usually transitory. But other uses of antibiotics exacerbate the resistance problem because they are inappropriate—namely, improper choice of antibiotic and length of application.

To make matters worse, the resistance genes, harbored in one

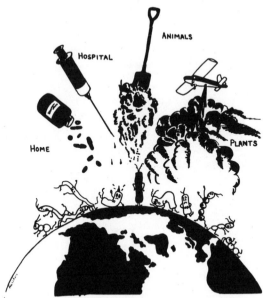

Figure 10.1. Antibiotics are used as therapeutic drugs in many different areas. The principal ones are for humans and for food-animal production, but another is agriculture. This usage includes home and hospital medications, growth promotant and therapeutic use in animals, and aerial treatments of plants and trees (Bonnie Marshall, Tufts University School of Medicine).

group of bacteria, can spread to vastly different types of bacteria and to areas far away. Resistant bacteria and their resistance genes do not need passports in order to cross country borders. They can quickly circumnavigate the globe, carried along as stowaways in humans, animals, and food products. This spread has been more rapid and insidious than anyone ever thought possible. Significantly, the resistant strains would have no survival advantage if there were no antibiotics present. Therefore, where use is limited, so are bacteria with resistance.

It is perhaps ironic and paradoxical that antibiotics, still the best agents for treating bacterial infections, are the single most important agents that select for and cause the propagation of bacteria resistant to them. This two-sided conflicting effect of these valuable drugs makes it crucial that we use them carefully.

Infectious disease experts have estimated that at least half of the human use of antibiotics in the United States, whether in the community at large or in hospitals, is unnecessary or inappropriate. Similar or higher levels of misuse have been documented in other parts of the world, but the actual extent of antibiotic misuse worldwide remains unknown. When this misuse is a superfluous use, there is an "extra" nontherapeutic selective force for the propagation of antibiotic resistant strains.

Today, antibiotic resistance thwarts our ability to cure diseases. The rise in multiresistance among bacteria, that is, the ability of a single disease-causing bacterium to resist more than one antibiotic, is steadily climbing to precarious proportions. An approach to curb this tide is sorely needed. Let us recapitulate how antibiotics are presently being used and how we can best allay their ability to encourage the emergence and spread of resistant strains.

AVAILABILITY TO THE CONSUMER

As noted before, in the United States and other industrialized nations, antibiotics for human treatment can be obtained only through prescription. This regulation is applied to protect individuals from misuse and causing potential harm to themselves. Despite the need for obtaining a doctor's prescription, there are ways to get prescription medication if one wants it, such as by coercing one's physician or hoarding leftover prescriptions. Rather than bother with throat cultures, which can be done in the office and speedily examined for "strep throat," some doctors simply hand out prescriptions. In many instances, especially when the patient has no fever, the problem may be viral, not bacterial, and the antibiotics are useless. Such physicians are not helping their patients, and they are certainly not helping society cope with a burgeoning worldwide resistance problem.

As we have seen, for the majority of the world's population, antibiotics are available over-the-counter in pharmacies, as easy to obtain as aspirin and cough medicines. The patient does not need to visit a physician, wait for a diagnosis, or get a prescription. If the antibiotic is carried in the local pharmacy, the consumer can obtain it; however, only the few who can afford the costs of these drugs can take advantage of their ready accessibility. For this latter reason, while it is theoretically possible for the majority of the population to have easy access to these drugs, most cannot buy them. In the Dominican Republic, for example, one day's treatment with ampicillin, a penicillin derivative, costs more than the daily wage of a typical farmworker.

Whatever the means of distribution, the common denominator of antibiotic usage in all countries is the individual consumer. Therefore, any attempt to improve the use of antibiotics must focus on the person who asks for, buys, and takes the antibiotic. We can make great strides toward curtailing side effects and curbing antibiotic resistance if we can convince individuals that these drugs are not "cure-alls." Each person should take an antibiotic only when needed, that is, only when suffering from a known bacterial infection. These drugs are not meant to treat symptoms—they are not to be taken at the first sign of a sore throat or cough. People should understand clearly why they should not be stockpiling antibiotics in their homes to be given out to other members of the family or to neighbors. Although antibiotics have been known and used for almost fifty years, people's attitudes toward them have changed very little. In the late 1950s, only twelve years after the success of penicillin and seven years after the discovery of the virtues of tetracycline and chloramphenicol, Henry Welch, then Director of the Division of Antibiotics of the U.S. Department of Health, Education and Welfare, stated in the New York Academy of Medicine's book, *The Impact of Antibiotics on Medicine and Society*:

The American public is like a huge sponge that absorbs antimicrobial agents like water, always eager to try the new one they have read about in their daily press or latest magazine, one whose miraculous cures emanated from the radio or television. It has reached the point where the physician can tell his patient—but he can not tell him much! The patient advises the doctor that he does not want antibiotic "A" because he has heard it is dangerous; he wants antibiotic "B" because a friend of his was cured with it. It makes no difference to him that his friend had an entirely unrelated infection. It's a "miracle drug"—let it perform its miracle.[1]

Has this opinion changed over these past thirty-plus years? Such an attitude has persisted into the present decade, and without some broad effort to change it, it will continue into the next decade and beyond. We are paying the price for such misconceptions now in the form of unnecessary side effects and rapidly increasing medical costs.

We need to reeducate ourselves—we, the antibiotic-consuming public. We must alter attitudes that have their origins in the initial discoveries of antibiotics and their timeworn label as "miracle drugs."

SOCIETAL CONSEQUENCES OF INDIVIDUAL MISUSE

Aside from the individual risks of side effects and allergies, there is a much larger societal effect stemming from widespread antibiotic use. This detrimental effect, however, is more subtle and certainly not one that is considered by the average individual who is taking the antibiotic. I am, of course, referring to the broad ecological changes that antibiotics produce. Antibiotic selection is environmental, not just individual, and the appearance and propagation of resistant forms of bacteria pose a serious threat to society at large. Selection of antibiotic resistant bacteria occurs in every user, wherever bacteria usually appear, such as in the

intestinal tract, the mouth, and on the skin. We accept this consequence if the antibiotic is medically needed, but if not, the change
in our bacterial flora is unnecessary and potentially harmful.
These resistant bacteria can move to family members and to other
people. While most of the resistant bacteria selected during antibiotic use are not those that cause harm to us, their resistance traits
are often transferable. These bacteria have the potential to pass
their resistant traits on to harmful bacteria with which they come
into contact.

A societal effect from antibiotics is set in motion every time
we inappropriately use these valuable drugs. As I stated in a
recent editorial, "Antibiotics are unique among pharmaceuticals in
that they treat populations as well as individuals. One's bacteria
are not solely one's own. Rather, they are shed, excreted, and otherwise spread into the environment, where they become part of a
common pool."[2] In fact, the individual's flora probably reflect the
environmental flora in which that person lives—the kinds of bacteria and the frequency of antibiotic resistance there (Figure 10.2).

A study that examined the frequency of antibiotic resistance
in intestinal *Escherichia coli* bacteria is pertinent to this point. The
investigators determined the numbers of resistant *E. coli* in the
feces of infants and small children in three geographically distant
cities on three different continents: Caracas, Venezuela; Qin Pu,
China; and Boston, Massachusetts.[3] The investigation unveiled a
number of important findings. First, in all three cities most of the
children being considered for the study groups had already received an antibiotic, even though most were under five years old.
Among the several hundred interviewed, fewer than 10% had not
taken an antibiotic, and this included a majority of infants. Focus-
ing on those children who had not received an antibiotic, the
examiners tested the amount of *E. coli* showing resistance to eight
separate drugs in their flora. In Boston, very few of this small
subgroup of infants had *E. coli* that were resistant to any of the
drugs; in those children who did, these resistant *E. coli* were
present in low numbers. This was not the case in the other two
cities. Here the flora of the infants showed large numbers of

resistant and multiresistant *E. coli*. Why the difference? The investigators have not yet fully solved the mystery, but one difference was clear from the outset of the study—antibiotics are obtained more easily and used more frequently in Venezuela and China than in Boston. These findings suggest that the total societal use of antibiotics may determine the native flora of each individual in that society, in the present case, these infants.

We can look into this question another way. Infants are born sterile, that is, without any bacteria. They have come from a sterile

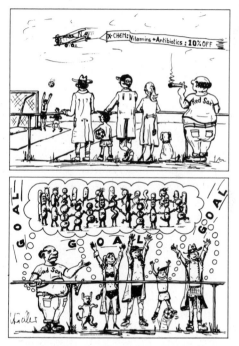

Figure 10.2. The bacteria associated with each individual may reflect common bacteria in the immediate environment and, in turn, society. Antibiotics can dramatically affect this societal microbiota (Herbert Hächler, University of Zurich, Zurich, Switzerland).

environment, namely, the womb of the mother. Once introduced into the environment, their bodies are quickly colonized by bacteria with which they have contact. This begins with the birthing room and the mother. These infants begin life without bacteria and without antibiotic resistance. They soon become colonized with the flora in their immediate environment. The relative frequency of resistant and susceptible forms of bacteria that they acquire at birth will depend on what is most frequent in that environment. They are, in a sense, barometers of their immediate bacterial "environment," *until* they begin taking antibiotics themselves. Once on antibiotics, they become part of a process of bacterial selection that will push the flora to even higher levels of resistance.

The authors of this *Escherichia coli* study proposed a goal for the future—a low resistance "index." If, as they showed, we start out life with low levels of bacterial resistance, let's strive to maintain this "resistance-free" state.[2] One clear goal is to reduce the reservoirs of resistance genes in the environment. And one way to do this is to improve the ways in which antibiotics are being used.

As soon as we entered the antibiotic era, microbiologists and clinicians began to notice bacterial resistance. The problem was first evident when penicillin-resistant staphylococci appeared in hospitals in England and subsequently were tabulated throughout the rest of the world. The full implications of resistance, however, were not realized until the last two decades. Seemingly overnight, doctors discovered that they could no longer cure common illnesses with conventional antibiotics. This problem was as evident in the general community as in the hospital, where children's acute ear infections, skin infections, and pneumonias remained unaffected by penicillins. Resistance traits had appeared in community-acquired bacteria that had previously been uniformly susceptible to antibiotics. This change was the direct consequence of the tremendous selective power of antibiotics for resistant types of bacteria. Additionally, there was the unexpected presence in the environment of genes already available to the microbial world that rendered bacteria resistant and that could be exchanged among them. Exacerbating this situation is the widespread attitude of the public. "So what if I take an antibiotic? What harm can it do?"

In most instances, this indirect consequence, that is, selection of a resistance trait or a resistant bacterium, may not affect a particular person at the time, but it potentially compromises the future antibiotic therapy of family members and neighbors. More directly, however, the ingestor can be put at risk. Patients under treatment for cancer, as we have noted, become more susceptible to infections and can contract diseases even from the normal bacteria colonizing their own skin and intestinal tracts. If these strains are resistant, even if they are not normally pathogenic, they can become life-threatening because of the patient's weakened condition, and because the resistance of these microorganisms circumvents treatment.

As people continue to misuse antibiotics, more resistant bacteria with different kinds of resistances are surfacing, and, in turn, newer and more expensive antibiotics are needed to treat them. We may reach a point where costs preclude availability. What will we do then? It is time for all of us to deal with the rising problem of resistance and correct the public's misconception about the all-encompassing power of antibiotics. We need to convince ourselves, and those seeking out these drugs, that antibiotics have a defined role in medical therapy and by taking them inappropriately we lay ourselves, as well as the rest of society, open to life-threatening risks.

WHO PROVIDES THE ANTIBIOTICS?

Putting the individual consumer aside for the moment, we should understand the role of the physicians, veterinarians, pharmacists, and government health officials who distribute these antibiotics. These prescribers represent a critical link in the chain leading from antibiotic production to antibiotic use and finally to antibiotic resistance. In developed countries, patients have little formal access to antibiotics without proper prescriptions. Thus, this group of prescribers holds the power to provide sound judgments in the dispersal of antibiotics. Yet, some will dispense antibiotics on demand by the patient or prescribe them as substitutes for other remedies that would have been just as effective and less risky. Antihistamines, fluids, and antiinflammatory agents are all that is needed for the relief of symptoms of the common cold.

In developing countries, however, such professional groups are not the primary dispensers of antibiotics. This role is often played by the local pharmacy. There are a number of reasons for this situation, not the least of which is the number of available physicians. While there is, on the average, one physician for every 520 people in developed countries, this number is about one to 2700 in most of the developing world, and the ratio can reach 17,000 patients per physician in the least developed countries. With so few physicians available, other ways of obtaining necessary drugs, including antibiotics, needed to be established. Thus, antibiotics are available through the pharmacy without a prescription or they can be bought through the black market. To some extent, the ease of procuring antibiotics relieves some of the problems created by the paucity of medical personnel for these people. Still, a safe balance between the health needs of the people and the efficacy of antibiotics must somehow be realized.

While over-the-counter sales have been one solution to the problem of too few doctors, the situation has created menacing results. The easy availability of antibiotics has contributed to the emergence and spread of resistant strains so that readily accessible drugs no longer cure common infections. Yet these antibiotics continue to be used. Consequently, rather than kill off the disease-causing agents, they enable them to thrive in the patient and spread easily to others. Money is wasted on ineffective medicines that could have been used to buy food or clothing.

Recently, a group from Nigeria, evaluating the rising frequency of antibiotic resistance there, spoke out on the need for newer antibiotics to treat common disease agents in the face of a high frequency of multidrug resistance to the older antibiotics. They explained,

> Health policies in most developing countries include some form of National Formulary leading to the purchase of a restricted range of drugs. In the case of antibacterials, this most likely means that the greater proportion of available funds is spent on the purchase of older and cheaper agents. But is this wise, in view of the high prevalence of strains that are now resistant to these agents? It undoubtedly looks sensible on the budget sheets, but would the average house-holder consider it a "good buy" if a new brand of detergent powder, marketed at one-third the price of other brands, carried a 60% or more chance that the packet contained sand instead of detergent? Probably not. And the same would seem to be true when older, cheaper antibiotics are given to patients without the sensitivity of the infecting organism being known. The householder would want to look inside the packet before it is purchased for use. Older antibiotics may be a waste of money, despite being cheap, unless it is also possible to "look inside the packet," by having facilities for bacteriological testing, before they are used.[4]

The same view was voiced by examiners of antibiotic use in Costa Rica.[5] Here, resistance to ampicillin, a penicillin derivative, in many Gram-negative pathogens was so high that the drug was hardly useful. The situation led to the removal of ampicillin from outpatient pharmacies and the addition of newer, albeit more expensive drugs to deal with these resistant microorganisms.

Given the poor health care delivery in developing countries, solutions are not easily envisioned, but some can and should be considered. For instance, certain antibiotics could be made available to the people by governments expressly to treat the major diseases or epidemics affecting that population. Acute respiratory tract bacterial infection is a common disease affecting infants and children in less developed countries. Treatment failure in this illness often means death. In making the choice of the right antibiotic, decision makers should know what the major disease agents are in their areas and what is the susceptibility of these bacteria to antibiotics. With this information, they could focus their limited budgets on just those particular antibiotics that are active against the recognized disease-causing agents known to exist in that region.

A limited number of drugs could thus be made available, namely those known to be effective for the disease at hand in a particular locale. Others, even the more expensive antibiotics, could be reserved for drastic problems of resistance. Such an approach would remove the need for supplying many different kinds of antibiotics. It would hold newer antibiotics in reserve that could be used to treat only those patients harboring otherwise untreatable antibiotic resistant infections. This approach would impart availability and effective use, despite limited public health monies in these countries. Such a rational system should bring more antibiotics, and, more significantly, the *right* ones, to areas where underuse and misuse of the drugs, *not* overuse, undermine medical therapy of the population.

UNDERUSE HAS UNFORTUNATE CONSEQUENCES

In the developing world, large numbers of people are at risk of dying from acute bacterial respiratory and gastrointestinal diseases, either because inadequate therapy is available or because whatever is available is not effective. Large numbers of appropriate antibiotics are needed to treat these individuals, who are often impoverished and unable to pay for a visit to a physician, let alone the cost of a course of antibiotics.

For many patients served in primary health care clinics in developing countries, a single dose of an antibiotic is all that is available or affordable. Paradoxically, this minimal treatment allows the illness to flourish. A study of antibiotic usage in a refugee camp on the Thai border, reported by a paramedic from the United States, illustrates this situation.[6] Over one-third of the patients received only a single antibiotic dose despite serious bacterial illnesses. The same paramedic also reported how antibiotics were stolen from local pharmacies and clinics and sold on the "black market" to people who could afford them and who then used them as they saw fit.

I personally have seen antibiotics, made attractive by their colorful capsules, sold in small plastic sacks in markets in Nairobi, Kenya. The source of these capsules and their effectiveness were not readily known. This kind of easy availability fosters gross misuse, which in turn propagates resistance and unsuccessful treatment both for the person and the community. In Bangladesh, as of 1990, over 80% of *Shigella dysenteriae* type 1, the cause of bloody diarrhea, were resistant to ampicillin or trimethoprim/sulfamethoxazole or both, agents of first choice in the treatment of this disease. Multidrug resistance was characteristic of *Shigella* of all types found there, as is also the situation in Vietnam, Africa, and South America. The leading culprit is not the antibiotic itself but its use or misuse. As one infectious disease expert explained, "Insufficient quantity or multiple antimicrobial agents are given simultaneously. Often antimicrobial agents are given when there is no indication for use."[7] How does this occur? As we discussed elsewhere, it is through easy availability in private pharmacies without the need for a physician's prescription (Figure 10.3).

In Southeast Asia, Latin America, and other less developed areas of the world, 70% to 80% of the patients who go to the local clinics have infectious disease problems that need antibiotic treatment. In a study conducted in Aceh Province in Indonesia in the mid-1980s, primary health care physicians reported that 65% of consecutive outpatients received or were prescribed antibiotics.[8] About a quarter of these patients purchased only half the amount of the antibiotic prescribed. This is, presumably, because of the high price they had to pay, along with the mistaken impression that just small amounts of these drugs were necessary to cure them of their diseases. In a similar analysis performed at about the same time, 70% of the patients attending an outpatient clinic in Santo Domingo, Dominican Republic, suffered from infectious diseases, predominantly caused by bacteria. Again, the economic constraints of the clinic gave the physicians there only enough

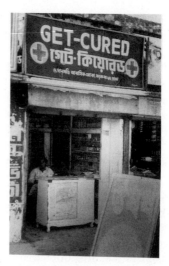

Figure 10.3. Over-the-counter sales in developing countries make antibiotics easily accessible to those who can afford them. This private pharmacy in Bangladesh claims to have the answer for all illnesses. It is this type of availability of antibiotics that many believe contributes largely to the propagation of resistant bacteria (Michael Bennish, Department of Medicine, New England Medical Center, Boston, Massachusetts).

antibiotic for the first day's treatment. The rest was to be filled by a prescription. About half of the patients never filled their prescription. They could not afford it. In all these examples, less than optimal antibiotic treatment is provided. This practice leads to failure to cure, as well as selection and propagation of resistant bacteria.

THE CRITICAL ROLE OF INDUSTRY

The pharmaceutical manufacturers play an integral role in the development and delivery of antibiotics. Most, if not all, of the major antibiotics currently in use have been developed through the auspices of the pharmaceutical industry. These companies had considerably fewer capital assets when they took on the development of penicillin in the early 1940s than they do now. That risky undertaking paid off and helped form the foundation of what is now a multibillion-dollar industry. Their efforts have brought major antibiotics into production and have made them available for the treatment of serious illnesses around the world. Like some physicians and other antibiotic dispensers who sometimes prescribe antibiotics inappropriately, however, the pharmaceutical industry has contributed to antibiotic misuse problems as well.

Marketing techniques for antibiotics made in one country that are then sold in another are often inconsistent, and, in some cases, are simply unethical. For example, some citations for antibiotics claim broader uses for people in one country than for people in another country. More importantly, all of the possible side effects are not listed on the package inserts in the antibiotic preparation. Many more precautions are listed for antibiotics sold in the United States than in less developed countries. Such inconsistencies have fostered unrest among consumer-based organizations that carefully examine products being introduced into their markets. When questioned, manufacturers often defend their actions by stating that they are only adhering to the regulations of the particular country. While this response may be true, consumer groups argue that this attitude is not ethical when dealing with human health. The problem here is that some countries are less demanding than others in these matters. The potential and severity of side effects should be printed on every drug label and provided as a standard in all countries, regardless of local regulations. The International Association of Pharmaceutical Companies advocates this principle, but discrepancies still exist. As a best case, it would seem fitting that the individual companies monitor their own practices.

Direct confrontation, legal actions, and the printed word from consumer organizations have brought these issues out into the open for the public to review. These consumer groups raise important questions and demand immediate answers. The groups include: Health Action International (HAI), which is an umbrella for many consumer organizations worldwide; the International Organization of Consumer Unions (IOCU); Social Audit in England; and the more recent Medical Lobby for Appropriate Marketing, Inc. The latter group has succeeded in getting several ineffective or potentially harmful drug combinations withdrawn. It has engineered the removal of drugs from certain combinations because they were superfluous and not useful. In other areas, misleading advertising claims have been modified. It is reassuring that, in many instances, industry representatives have responded to these queries either by explaining their rationale, removing or altering the product, or changing the package insert description.

THE COST, TO SOCIETY AND THE INDIVIDUAL, OF ANTIBIOTIC RESISTANCE

Certainly the most critical consequence of antibiotic resistance is the compromised therapy of human disease. Another mounting and disturbing consequence of resistance, however, revolves around the price tag for treatment. Someone must pay for the higher costs of newer drugs that are needed to combat resistant bacteria. Medical insurance companies, the government, and the individual now face, and will continue to face, higher and higher prices for the new antibiotics being developed to treat the multiresistant forms of bacterial disease. Some of these drugs can cost over $500 a day for treatment! Consider that price next to a cost of less than a dollar a day for some older forms of penicillin. One investigation from the United States Centers for Disease Control reviewed 175 published and unpublished accounts of hospital- and community-acquired bacterial infections. They concluded that, for infections in the hospital and the community, "The mortality, the likelihood of hospitalization and the length of hospital stay were usually at least twice as great for patients infected with drug-resistant strains as for those infected with drug-susceptible strains of the same bacteria."[9] The inability to treat effectively a resistant infection immediately in an elderly patient may mean a greater chance of death than if the bacteria were susceptible; the same for a child. Timing is important in the struggle between the patient and the bacteria's ability to overwhelm him or her.

Another study used different mathematical models and assumptions to arrive at the actual costs of resistance to society. Depending on whether or not death was a consequence, the total societal costs of antibiotic resistance ranged from $150 million (without deaths) to $3 billion (with deaths) each year in the United States alone.[10] This study tried to factor in, as well, the effect of a resistant infectious agent appearing in one year on the cost to society in later years.

In developing countries of the world, the additional costs for new medication cannot possibly be met and, thus, these new, more costly antibiotics are not available there. Individuals living in the developed world are also fortunate in having excellent public health conditions that curb the incidence and spread of infectious diseases. Most of them have the ability to pay the higher price of newer drugs when faced with antibiotic resistance. This option is not open to the less fortunate people living in developing, and often more populous, areas of the world. We must also consider the cost to the pharmaceutical companies of developing new antibiotics to treat these resistant bacteria. Millions of dollars are invested in the discovery, development, and animal and human testing of new antibiotics. This procedure takes years—a mean of ten years—as well as great sums of money. We have neither the time nor the money to spare. These mounting monetary and time constraints have provoked some companies to abandon the field of antibiotic research altogether—a decision that poses further detriments to society. Once tested and approved, an antibiotic enters the market. Herein lies the conflict between research, development, and marketing. The company, its board members and stockholders, want to recuperate their investment, the sooner the better in this competitive field. To do so, the new antibiotic must be advertised to physicians and sold in pharmacies. How much of the cost should be returned in the first year? The second year? If there is concern about an upcoming, competitive drug, the pressure to sell as much as possible, as soon as possible, will be heightened immediately. No one can blame the pharmaceutical sales agents for encouraging the use of their product—within reason. The control on its choice and usage, however, must be at the level of the consumer (hospital pharmacy, government health officer, health plan officer) and prescriber. If the medical need is met by the new drug and the advantages over older, less expensive, agents are clear, then the new drug should be purchased and used. Yet, where less expensive older agents can be used, would it not be wiser to use these? While the pharmaceutical house may receive less revenue in a single year, the time between drug introduction and the emergence of resistant bacteria will be decreased. This will provide the pharmaceutical company with a longer "run" for the product. And the cost to the entire health care industry will be lessened.

PROBLEMS IN THE DEVELOPING WORLD

The numbers of people in the United States suffering from the consequences of antibiotic resistance are small when compared with the much larger numbers of people in less developed nations who become infected with common resistant pathogens, those causing diarrhea or pneumonia. None of us who has followed the resistance problem will forget the thousands of lives lost in Central America in the 1970s when a multiresistant *Shigella* could not be touched with the available antibiotics. Resistance was still a curiosity and the consequence was brought home clearly in this epidemic. Some physicians were convinced they were dealing with an amoebic parasite causing the diarrhea—they had never been confronted with such a resistant bacterium. The more recent epidemic of dysentery in Zaire in the early 1980s was also caused by a multiresistant *Shigella dysenteriae*. Hundreds lost their lives from an infection that should have ordinarily responded to antibiotics and fluid therapy. Such a situation could conceivably emerge in the developed world, if we continue on our present path. Let us not forget the problem with multiresistant staphylococci in the hospitals of Melbourne, Australia.

THE ANIMAL ISSUE

The use of antibiotics as growth-promoting agents in livestock has generated heated controversy in the United States and Europe for several decades. Whereas Europe responded in the 1970s by banning any antibiotics being used for humans from being used in feed additives, the United States Food and Drug Administration has not. The Natural Resources Defense Council, whose mandate includes wide environmental issues, adopted the animal feed problem as one of its investigational issues during the 1980s. It filed legal briefs with the Food and Drug Administration, including its famous 1985 "Imminent Hazard" petition that it placed before Margaret Heckler, then Secretary of Health and Human Services. This latter document pointed to a large number of deaths from *Salmonella* infections linked to animal products, and associated the effect of antibiotic usage at any level with the emergence of resistant *Salmonella*. Margaret Heckler rejected the petition on the basis of lack of evidence for an "imminent" hazard, but, quoting Frank Young, the FDA Commissioner, she allowed the possibility of the issue to be resolved when more data had been accumulated.

The issue did, in fact, eventually, come before a committee formed by the National Academy of Sciences' Institute of Medicine a few years later. This highly esteemed group of experts examined only the risk of death from use of antibiotics in animal feed. Because of limited data on other microorganisms, they focused on *Salmonella* as the causative agent. Thus, they left out the general issue of morbidity and the specific consequences of other disease-causing agents such as *Listeria* or *Campylobacter* or even *Escherichia coli*. This group, reviewing past and new data, concluded that although the committee was "unable to find a substantial body of direct evidence that established the existence of a definite human health hazard in the use of subtherapeutic concentrations of penicillin and the tetracyclines in the animal feeds . . . [nevertheless] the committee believes that there is indirect evidence implicating subtherapeutic use of antimicrobials in producing resistance in infectious bacteria that cause a potential health hazard.[11] But they were unable to assign a clear value factor to the risk. This inexactitude stems from the inability to assess which kind of use, therapeutic or growth-promoting, led to the emergence and propagation of resistant bacteria. The United States FDA is still sitting on its decision of whether or not to eliminate this kind of antibiotic use. Nothing is being done actively in the interim. Antibiotics are still fed to animals while the experts study the numbers.

We expect that the debate on the use of antibiotics for growth promotion will continue to be discussed as more data are accrued. Perhaps, as we are now seeing, the issue will die out because farmers are voluntarily withdrawing antibiotics and replacing them with nonantibiotic alternatives or other more natural farming methods. The public has become a powerful lobby—asking for meat and agricultural products that are untainted by antibiotics or other chemicals.

RESISTANCE VIEWED FROM THE WORLD PERSPECTIVE

The problem of resistance is multifaceted in its origins and manifestations, but we can still surmount it. Although resistance is clearly an international problem and the demographics of language and mentality may be different in each country, there are similarities in the profiles of all members of society prescribing and consuming antibiotics everywhere. It is the relative numbers of each antibiotic using/prescribing societal type that may be different, depending on the country and its number of medical personnel. The universal features of this widespread problem have convinced individuals and groups in countries worldwide to take an active role in solving it. Countries on all continents are becoming increasingly aware that antibiotic resistance is not a problem unique to their country or even their continent. There need be no embarrassment that resistance has emerged in their country—bacterial resistance is a global dilemma.

A group of over 100 experts from more than 30 countries throughout the world concluded a three-year project in 1986 sponsored by the Fogarty International Center of the United States National Institutes of Health.[12] This group took a critical and comprehensive look at the state of antibiotic usage and antibiotic resistance worldwide. They found that almost enough antibiotics are being made in the world today to meet the present needs of the world's population, that is, if all antibiotics were effective and resistance were not a deterrent. These conditions, however, are not present and the distribution of these antibiotics is highly unequal. In the developed world, antibiotics are plentiful. In areas of the world where they are sorely needed, antibiotics are available only in limited supply. Yet these are the areas with the highest frequency of infectious diseases. The reason for this hazardous health situation is poor public sanitation, in particular with regard to the water supply. To make matters worse, these are the same areas where antibiotic resistance poses the greatest threat to the population. Translated into public health parlance, this situation means more spread of disease and more resistance.

This study also found that the frequency of resistance to some of the most common antibiotics had reached high levels among certain bacterial populations of individual countries where they appeared to persist. This finding meant that, although enough total antibiotics were being produced to cover the world, a good part of these antibiotics would not be useful in the face of large-scale resistance. The levels of resistance varied by antibiotic and by country. The reasons for these differences were not clear, but could and should certainly take into account differences in patterns of antibiotic use, or differences in public health measures. Addressing this point have been studies that showed a vastly different country-to-country utilization of antibiotics and even the phenomenon of different quantities being administered in hospitals within the same country. For instance, in Japan, cephalosporin use per person was more than ten times that in Sweden and Australia and four to five times that in most other countries. To a great extent, this larger consumption in Japan was attributed to a financial gain received by the physician prescribing the cephalosporins. On the other hand, a financial incentive cannot explain the twofold difference found in the consumption of certain antibiotics in eight hospitals in Sweden.[13] That this kind of difference should exist in Sweden, where the diseases, geography, and the people are so homogeneous, indicates that other factors are influencing decisions about antibiotic use. These differences must lie in the rationale behind the decision-makers themselves, specifically, the physicians controlling the treatment. Understanding the reasons for different antibiotic utilization rates in Sweden and elsewhere would help to develop a plan to match the availability of antibiotics with the needs of a country.

The Fogarty Task Force study found that, while resistance to particular antibiotics varied greatly with the microorganisms, still, overall, countries far apart shared the same kinds of resistant strains of bacteria even if their frequencies were different. Today, worldwide, about 30–50% of all *E. coli* commonly involved in urinary tract infections are resistant to penicillin drugs, tetracyclines, and other common antibiotics. Fortunately, we have other drugs on hand to treat these resistant infections. A more diverse range of resistance frequencies is found for *Hemophilus influenzae*, which can cause ear infections, meningitis, and pneumonia. Here a resistance frequency range of 10–90% is noted to ampicillins, tetracyclines, and up to five different antibiotics, depending on the geographical location.

The Fogarty study further showed that each country of the world was dealing with the resistance problem at a somewhat different societal level. The more industrialized countries of North America and Europe were dealing with diseases of resistant and multiresistant bacteria among individuals in particular communities or in hospitals. Most infectious diseases in the United States affect an individual or, at most, his or her family. On a rare occasion, larger groups have been infected, such as when epidemics of gastrointestinal diseases have hit schools and nurseries. In the late 1980s, an epidemic of multiresistant *Shigella* causing diarrhea plagued two Indian reservations in the United States. Once again, alternative antibiotics and public health measures succeeded in curbing the outbreaks before they reached dangerous proportions. Unfortunately, this kind of successful outcome is not seen commonly in the developing world. Here, resistant bacteria often thwart treatment of large numbers of patients in many countries. The reason—inadequate public health measures to curb the spread of the infectious agents.

Despite the lower numbers afflicted by infectious disease, the developed world has its own share of serious resistance problems. In the United States, for instance, the treatment of common community infections, such as ear infections, gonorrheal infections, and pneumonias, is gravely thwarted by resistance to penicillins and tetracyclines.

PERSISTENCE OF RESISTANCE

While we know that antibiotic usage has contributed to the selection of resistance genes, we do not understand what causes the sustained, relatively high levels of these resistances in areas and countries where the antibiotic has been stopped. Since this persistence is not associated with the constant presence of an antibiotic, it presumably relates to other features of the resistance phenomenon. We also know that there is a slow loss from the environment of antibiotic resistance determinants, once selected.

To understand the phenomenon, we should take a look at the total picture. It is clear that, after a period of antibiotic selection, there exists a resident population of bacteria that harbors resistance genes. These bacteria are not very different from the other bacteria usually found in these environmental niches, except that they bear resistance genes. When the antibiotic is removed, these bacteria remain because they have now become a major component of the normal microbial flora. There is no factor or agent selecting *against* the resistant bacteria. These features probably contribute to the persistence of these genes in bacteria normally resident in that ecological niche.

But there may be other contributing factors. Many resistant bacteria also carry genes for resistance to heavy metals, such as mercury. Recent evidence suggests that mercury is a common environmental contaminant.[14] This fact may be especially true in the human body, where tooth fillings bearing mercury are almost universally present and from which small amounts of mercury are released on a daily basis. Enough mercury predictably flows through the intestine to select for mercury-resistant bacterial strains. If these strains also bear antibiotic resistance genes on the same plasmid or in the same bacteria as those with mercury resistance, then the mercury serves to maintain antibiotic as well as mercury resistance in that environment and in these bacteria. In other words, one growth-inhibiting agent, in this case mercury, can select for mercury-resistant bacteria that carry resistance to other growth-inhibiting agents, namely antibiotics. All the resistances have found their way into the same bacteria and often onto the same plasmid. This is the same phenomenon we discussed before in regard to one antibiotic being able to select for plasmids with resistance to other antibiotics.

INTERNATIONAL RESPONSE TO ANTIBIOTIC
AVAILABILITY AND RESISTANCE

How does the world community deal with resistance on one hand and antibiotic availability on the other? The World Health Organization has convened many groups of experts to look into the problem, to identify the factors causing resistance, and to find the correct means of dealing with this issue. Their findings, recorded in a number of publications, emphasize that antibiotics are the primary selective agents for resistance and so their usage, whether too little or too much, must be evaluated and improved. Underlying these reports was the apparent need for national efforts to be carried out by local individuals working in concert with government authorities, to deal with the problem at the local level.

All reports stress that one country cannot dictate to another country how to distribute or control the use of antibiotics, but a general plan could be derived to help stem the tide of antibiotic resistance. This growing problem requires a universal effort, with all countries working together toward a common end, similar to recent world forums on global warming and fishing rights. At a minimum, certain guidelines can be drawn based on current scientific information. These guidelines can focus on antibiotic use and the existence of resistance. The kinds of bacteria causing the most common diseases should be identified in each country. Their susceptibility to antibiotics should be made well-known. Then, appropriate antibiotics can be purchased, distributed, and used effectively in that particular country. It is important to remember, however, that every country is connected through the microbial network. The antibiotic needs of each country should be met, but cautious and discriminate use must be practiced every-where since every human being's health is at stake. Otherwise, the single country's efforts will be fraught with failure as new forms of resistant microorganisms travel across national and international borders.

The need for a major international cooperative effort has evolved from the conclusions of the expert groups for the World Health Organization and others. But until 1981 there was still no organized channel for communicating local situations to international audiences. The need arose for a consortium, an alliance, of concerned people worldwide to deal with the issue from the grassroots level—from those using and prescribing these drugs on up to heads of state. Such an organization arose as a result of a conference in the Dominican Republic in January 1981.

Over 200 participants from developing as well as developed countries came to a meeting in Santo Domingo to discuss the medical problems and ecology of resistance genes and their transferable vehicles—the plasmids. What emerged was a recognition that antibiotic resistance was not just the affliction of particular nations, but was global. The meeting put aside taboos about talking about the problem; it revealed that antibiotic resistance was worldwide and manifest in different ways in different countries. The overall message was clear—antibiotics were being misused, everywhere.

The participants realized a need to get this message across to the public—to remove the constraints on talking about the problem and to let people know its extent before it was really too late to do anything about it. Only open discussion among nations could help control this mounting, now fully evident public health menace.

Out of this meeting came an "Antibiotic Misuse Statement" that was endorsed by hundreds of clinicians, researchers, and scientific societies worldwide. It declared, "We are faced with a worldwide public health problem," and went on to discuss antibiotic resistance and the major ways it was being propagated.

The statement was translated into many languages including French, Spanish, Italian, Portuguese, Chinese, and Russian. It was formally presented at press conferences that took place simultaneously on August 4, 1981 in Boston, Massachusetts; Santo Domingo, Dominican Republic; Mexico City, Mexico; and São Paulo, Brazil (Figure 10.4).

The public responded with a flurry of questions and concern.

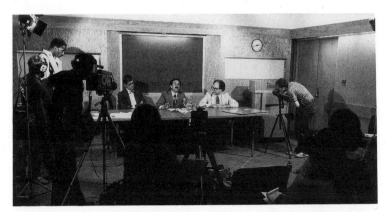

Figure 10.4. On August 4, 1981, pursuant to discussions about antibiotic misuse and resistance worldwide at a meeting in Santo Domingo, Dominican Republic, investigators in four cities worldwide presented an Antibiotic Misuse Statement. With the author (center) (Dr. Levy) at this press conference in Boston were Dr. George Jacoby (left) of Harvard University Medical School and the Massachusetts General Hospital, and Nobel Laureate Dr. Walter Gilbert (right) of Harvard University (Photo Department, Tufts University School of Medicine).

To most, this was news—disconcerting news. *Newsweek* and *Time* magazines featured the statement and its message in their medical news of the week. Articles and editorials appeared in the *New York Times*, the *Washington Post* and newspapers throughout the world. The response was dramatic and, more importantly, international. The scientific journal, *Nature*, featured an entire page-long editorial entitled "Saving antibiotics from themselves." The statement of misuse served its initial purpose, to make the world aware of the gravity of the problem and its global presence.

THE ALLIANCE FOR THE PRUDENT USE OF ANTIBIOTICS (APUA)

APUA emerged from this meeting and its subsequent resolution. This internationally-based group, whose present membership extends to more than 80 countries of the world, communicates basic tenets of proper antibiotic usage and the problems of antibiotic resistance to its members through a regular quarterly newsletter and various notices and forms of correspondence (Figure 10.5). It is the only organization of its kind, dedicated solely to the improved use and knowledge about a therapeutic product, not a disease. Its rationale is that antibiotics are crucial to all medical therapies involving people of all ages—in medicine, pediatrics, and surgery—and must be safeguarded vigilantly. Countries such as Bangladesh, Australia, China, Guatemala, and Venezuela have formed groups or APUA chapters to deal with the issue locally. Other chapters are currently in the planning stage. Through

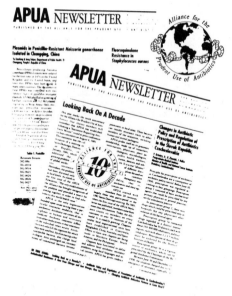

Figure 10.5. The Alliance for the Prudent Use of Antibiotics, established at the end of 1981, has members from over 80 countries worldwide. Through communication and education, APUA advocates appropriate use of antibiotics (APUA, Boston, Massachusetts).

communication and education, the organization seeks to promote improved use of antibiotics and to protect their long-term efficacy.

In order to be effective, APUA acts outside of political and economic pressures. Its members are individuals, doctors, dentists, pharmacists, veterinarians, biologists, microbiologists, public health officials, and others whose professions include handling antibiotics directly or confronting resistance in the home, hospital, or laboratory. This international group is making people all over the world cognizant of the resistance problem. It conveys the equally important message that antibiotic availability is important for disease eradication, not to be curtailed just when resistant variants appear. In many countries, this means making antibiotics *more* available, not *less* available, while adhering to effective doses.

Communication and cooperation between all nations is necessary to win the battle against the looming problem of resistance. Although one country can maintain strict adherence to better policies of antibiotic use, it would still run the risk of picking up and propagating resistant strains from other countries that are not so diligent. Through prudent usage, a resistant pathogen arising in one country could be contained in the country of origin and successfully eliminated before it has the chance to spread to the rest of the world. Everyone concerned will admit that it is a slow process, but giant steps do occur, such as the removal of fixed combinations of antibiotics in Spain and the greatly improved antibiotic usage in Australia and Brazil. What each country needs is support from its government in order to establish an antibiotic policy, an achievable reality in the wake of a global effort.

GOALS FOR THE DECADE

It is inappropriate to point a finger at any one particular participant using or dispensing antibiotics as the cause of the resistance problem. As noted earlier, antibiotic use is pervasive in our society. In each phase of antibiotic production, prescription, and use, there are some people who act responsibly and some who do not. An understanding must be reached in each area in order to see that inappropriate usage is curtailed. When incorrect use or faulty prescriptions persist despite medical and public opinion, actions should be taken to deal vigorously with the offenders. This response, as we mentioned before, can come directly only from local medical authorities. The most effective group, in the United States at least, is the prepay medical systems that monitor both patient use and physician prescribing profiles. If users and prescribers agree to look at their usage patterns more carefully, then industry members should also ascribe importance to seeing that their products are used rationally and effectively. The economics of the issue cannot be brushed aside, but then, there is no evidence that good and ethical practices will bring lower profits.

The goal in the next decade and, we hope before the year 2000, is to make antibiotics more available in the areas where they are most needed and to discourage frivolous use in areas where they are currently being overused. Education must remove the false impressions and attitudes about these drugs in the minds of the consumer and the prescriber. All concerned groups should carefully examine the factors that cause the emergence of resistance and help curtail these resistant strains as they appear in one country or another. It is efforts such as those displayed by the Fogarty International Center, the World Health Organization, and APUA that are bringing global attention to the fact that resistant bacteria are a continuing problem. It is these and other groups yet to be formed who may help conquer this impending threat. But they need the support of the world population—consumers and prescribers alike.

The resistance gene pool is constantly multiplying, as are the numbers of microorganisms resistant to more than one antibiotic. If we ignore the problem, single-drug therapy will simply become obsolete. Our goal should be to attempt to maintain the efficacy of the antibiotics we have by determining which diseases they can still eradicate and which microorganisms are still largely susceptible. We should develop new antibiotics and use them appro-

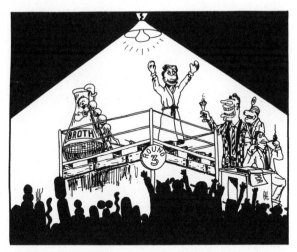

Figure 10.6. Mankind wins the next round. Through concerted efforts on the part of everyone developing, dispensing, and consuming antibiotics, humans can emerge victorious in their struggles with the microbial world (Herbert Hächler, University of Zurich, Zurich, Switzerland).

priately (Figure 10.6). Studies that reveal the basis for resistance should be encouraged and supported. These could lead to the rational design of new drugs or special drug treatments that are not subjected to the resistance mechanism. At the same time, we should put into action a new public-awareness model for the use of antibiotics that will protect the new drugs from becoming rapidly outdated through the same resistance problems. This kind of commitment should move us towards using antibiotics more wisely, more efficiently, and more appropriately. We could then control the rise in antibiotic resistance and assure the success of antibiotics now and for generations to come.

REFERENCES CITED

CHAPTER 1

1. The *Boston Sunday Globe*, November 29, 1942.
2. The *Boston Herald*, November 29, 1942.
3. The *Boston Daily Globe*, November 30, 1942.
4. The *Boston Daily Globe*, December 2, 1942.
5. The *New York Times*, p. 21, June 26, 1945.

CHAPTER 2

1. Waksman, S. A. The microbiology of soil and the antibiotics. In: *The Impact of the Antibiotics on Medicine and Society*. (Galdston, I., Ed.) International Universities Press, Inc. New York, p. 3, 1958.
2. Cowen, D. L. and Segelman, A. B. *Antibiotics in Historical Perspective*. Merck Sharp and Dohme International, Rahway, NJ, 1981.

CHAPTER 3

1. Ebbell, B. *The Papyrus Ebers*. Lewin and Munksgaard, Copenhagen, 1937.

2. Contenau, G. *La Médicine en Assyrie et en Babylone*. Librairie Maloine, Paris, 1938.
3. Walsh, J. J. *The Popes and Science*. Fordham University Press, New York. Appendix III (translation provided in *J. Amer. Med. Assoc.*, January 1908), pp. 419–423, 1911.
4. Guerra, F. *American Medical Bibliography 1639–1783*. Lathrop C. Harper Inc., New York, 1962.
5. Theobold, J. *Every Man His Own Physician*, Third Edition. London, 1764.

CHAPTER 5

1. Cohen, D., Creek, G., and Sayers, R. *Haemophilus influenzae* infections in American children living in the U.K. *Lancet i*:101, 1982.

CHAPTER 6

1. Pritchard, W. R. and Loew, F. M., Veterinary Medicine: Looking toward the 21st century. In: *Perspectives on the Health Professions*. Chapter 1. (O'Neil, E. H., Ed.). Pew Health Professions Programs, Duke University, 1990.

CHAPTER 9

1. *La Revue Prescrire* p. 2, April, 1984.
2. Hook, E. H., Brady, W. E., Reichart, C. A. *et al.* Determinants of emergence of antibiotic-resistant *Neisseria gonorrhoeae*. *J. Infect. Dis. 159*:900–906.
3. Nelson, W. L., Kennedy, D. L., Lao, C. S., and Kuritsky, J. N. Outpatient systemic antiinfective use by children in the United States, 1977–1986. *Pediat. Infect. Dis. J. 7*:505–509, 1988.
4. Reves, R. R., Fong, M., Pickering, L. K. *et al.* Risk factors for fecal colonization with trimethoprim-resistant and multiresistant *Escherichia coli* among children in day-care centers in Houston, Texas. *Antimicrob. Agents Chemother. 34*:1429–1434, 1990.
5. Corpet, D. E. Antibiotic resistance from food. *N. Engl. J. Med. 318*:1206–1207, 1988.
6. Wang, F. and Tai, T-Y. People's Republic of China: clinical antibiotic use. *APUA Newsletter 4*:4:1, 7, 1986.

CHAPTER 10

1. Welch, H. Antibiotics 1943–1955: Their development and role in present-day society. In: *The Impact of Antibiotics on Medicine and Society*, (Galdston, I., Ed.). International Universities Press, Inc. New York, p. 85, 1958.
2. Levy, S. B. Starting life resistance-free. *N. Engl. J. Med.* 323:335–337, 1990.
3. Lester, S. C., del Pilar Pla, M., Wang, F. *et al.* The carriage of *Escherichia coli* resistant to antimicrobial agents by healthy children in Boston, in Caracas, Venezuela and in Qin Pu, China. *N. Engl. J. Med.* 323:285–289, 1990.
4. Montefiore, D. G., Rotimi, V. O., and Adeyeme-Doro, O. Antibiotic resistance in Nigeria: impact on drug choice. *APUA Newsletter* 9:2:1, 6–8, 1991.
5. Lee, D. Changing antibiotic utilization patterns in Costa Rica. *APUA Newsletter* 9:1:7–8, 1991.
6. Macauley, C. Antibiotic usage in an outpatient clinic—Thailand 1984. *APUA Newsletter* 3:4:4–5, 1985.
7. Bennish, M. Increasing resistance among *Shigella* isolates in Bangladesh: will a rational use drug policy help? *APUA Newsletter* 9:4:6–7, 1991.
8. Azof, A., Solter, S. Mizan, M., and Hamed, A. F. Antibiotic use; Aceh Province, Indonesia. *APUA Newsletter* 4:3:1,6, 1986.
9. Holmberg, S. D., Solomon, S. L. and Blake, P. A., Health and economic impacts of antimicrobial resistance. *Rev. Infect. Dis.* 9:1065–1078, 1987.
10. Phelps, C. E. Bug/Drug Resistance. *Medical Care* 27:194–203, 1989.
11. Swartz *et al.* Human health risks with the subtherapeutic use of penicillins or tetracyclines in animal feed, National Academy Press, Washington, D.C., p. 194, 1989.
12. Levy, S. B., Burke, J., and Wallace, E. (Eds.). Antibiotic use and antibiotic resistance worldwide. *Rev. Infect. Dis.* 9:Suppl 3, 1987
13. Jansson, C. and Skold, O. Variations on the use of antibiotics among Swedish hospitals. *APUA Newsletter* 8:1:2–3, 1990.
14. Summers, A. O., Vimy, M., and Lorscheider, F. "Silver" dental fillings provoke an increase in mercury and antibiotic resistant bacteria in the mouth and intestines of primates. *APUA Newsletter* 9:3:4–5, 1991.

BIBLIOGRAPHY

Cope, O. Care of the victims of the Cocoanut Grove fire at the Massachusetts General Hospital. *N. Engl. J. Med.* 229:138–147, 1943.

Hobby, G. L. *Penicillin Meeting the Challenge.* Yale University Press, New Haven, 1989.

Macionis, J. Boston's nightclub tragedy (1942). *Inferno*, pp. 147–163, 1967.

Sheehan, J. and Ross, R. N. The fire that made penicillin famous. *Yankee Magazine*, pp. 125–203, 1982.

CHAPTER 2

Abraham, E. P., Chain, E., Fletcher, C. M. *et al.* Further observations on penicillin. *The Lancet*, pp. 177–188, August 16, 1941.

Chain, E., Florey, H. W., Gardner, A. D. *et al.* Penicillin as a chemotherapeutic agent. *The Lancet*, pp. 226–228, August 24, 1940.

Fleming, A. On the antibacterial action of cultures of a *Penicillium*, with special reference to their use in the isolation of *B. influenzae*. *Brit. J. Exp. Path.* 10:226–236, 1929.

Fleming, A. (Ed.) *Penicillin: Its Practical Application.* Butterworths and Co. Ltd. London, 1946.

Florey, H. W. The use of micro-organisms for therapeutic purposes. *Brit. Med. J.*, pp. 635–642, November 10, 1945.

Gray, G. W. Antibiosis. *Scientific American*, pp. 27–34, August, 1944.

Life magazine, pp. 58–59, July 17, 1944.

MacFarlane, G. *Alexander Fleming. The Man and the Myth.* Harvard University Press, Cambridge, 1984.

Moburg, C. L. and Cohn, Z. A. (Eds.) *Launching the Antibiotic Era.* The Rockefeller University Press, New York, 1990.

Pasteur, L. La theorie des germes et ses applications à la medecine et à la chirugie. Oeuvres de Pasteur. *C. R. Acad. Sci.* LXXXVI, April 29, 1878.

Sedillot, C., De l'influence des decouvertes de M. Pasteur sur les progres de la chirugie. *C. R. Acad. Sci.* LXXXVI, p. 634–640, 1878.

Time magazine, pp. 61–68, May 15, 1944.

Vuillemin, P. Antibiose et symbiose. *C. R. Assoc. Fr. Acad. Sci.* 2:525–543. Seance du 14 aout, 1889.

CHAPTER 3

Bryan, C. P. *The Papyrus Ebers.* Geoffrey Blis, London, 1930.

Buchan, W. *Domestic Medicine or the Family Physician.* Royal College of Physicians, Edinburgh, 2nd American edition, Philadelphia, 1774.

Garrison, F. H. *Introduction to the History of Medicine.* Fourth edition. W. B. Saunders, Philadelphia, 1929.

Gordon, B. L. *Medicine Throughout Antiquity.* F. A. Davis Co., Philadelphia, 1949.

Guthrie, D. *A History of Medicine.* Thomas Nelson and Sons Ltd., New York, 1945.

Inglis, B. *A History of Medicine.* World Publishing Company, Cleveland, 1965.

Majno, G. *The Healing Hand: Man and Wound in the Ancient World.* Harvard University Press, Cambridge, MA, 1975.

Moir, D. M. *Outlines of the Ancient History of Medicine.* William Blakewood, Edinburgh, 1831.

Netter, W., transl. of Peters, H. *Pictorial History of Ancient Pharmacy and Medicine.* Engelhard & Co., Chicago, 1889.

CHAPTER 4

Chow, J. W., Fine, M. J., and Shlaes, D. M. *Enterobacter* bacteremia: clinical features and emergence of antibiotic resistance during therapy. *Ann. Int. Med.* 115:585–590, 1991.

Croft, B. A. Arthropod resistance to insecticides: a key to pest control failures and successes in North American apple orchards. *Ent. Exp. Appl. 31*:88–110, 1982.

Datta, N., Faiers, M. C., Reeves, D. S. *et al.* R factors in *Escherichia coli* in faeces after oral chemotherapy in general practice. *The Lancet ii*: 312–315, 1971.

Davis, C. D. and Anandan, J. The evolution of R factor: a study of a "preantibiotic" community in Borneo. *N. Engl. J. Med. 282*:117–122, 1970.

Deuchars, K. L. and Ling, V. P-glycoprotein and multidrug resistance in cancer chemotherapy. *Sem. Oncology 16*:156–165, 1989.

Gardner, P., Smith, D. H., Beer, H., and Moellering, R. C., Jr. Recovery of resistance (R) factors from a drug-free community. *The Lancet*, pp. 774–776, October 11, 1969.

George, A. M. and Levy, S. B. Amplifiable resistance to tetracycline, chloramphenicol, and other antibiotics in *Escherichia coli*: identification of a non-plasmid mediated efflux system for tetracycline. *J. Bacteriol. 155*:531–540, 1983.

Hughes, V. M. and Datta, N. Conjugative plasmids in bacteria of the "preantibiotic" era. *Nature 302*:725–726, 1983.

Kloos, W. E. Effect of single antibiotic therapy on *Staphylococcus* community structure. *APUA Newsletter 5*:4:1–2, 1987.

Krogstad, D. J., Schlesinger, P. H., and Herwaldt, B. L. Antimalarial agents: mechanisms of chloroquine resistance. *Antimicrob. Agents Chemother. 32*:799–801, 1988.

Levy, S. B. Microbial resistance to antibiotics: an evolving and persistent problem. *The Lancet i*:83–88, 1982.

Levy, S. B. Evolution and spread of tetracycline resistance determinants. *J. Antimicrob. Chemother. 24*:1–3, 1989.

Levy, S. B. and Miller, R. V. Eds. *Gene Transfer in the Environment.* McGraw-Hill Publishing Co., New York, 1989.

Levy, S. B., Marshall, B., Schluederberg, S. *et al.* High frequency of antimicrobial resistance in human fecal flora. *Antimicrob. Agents Chemother. 32*: 1801–1806, 1988.

Mare, I. J. Incidence of R factors among gram-negative bacteria in drug-free human and animal communities. *Nature* (London) *220*:1046–1047, 1968.

Mare, I. J. and Coetzee, J. N. The incidence of transmissible drug resistance factors among strains of *Escherichia coli* in the Pretoria area. *S.A. Med. J.*, pp. 980–981, November 5, 1966.

Moller, J. K., Bak, A. L., Stenderup, A., Zachariae, H., and Afzelius, H. Changing patterns of plasmid-mediated resistance during tetracycline therapy. *Antimicrob. Agents Chemother. 11*:388–391, 1977.

Murray, B. E., Renismer, E. R., and DuPont, H. L. Emergence of high-level trimethoprim resistance in fecal *Escherichia coli* during oral administration of trimethoprim or trimethoprim-sulfamethoxazole. *N. Engl. J. Med. 306*:130–135, 1982.

Novick, R. P. Penicillinase plasmids of *Staphylococcus aureus. Fed. Proc. 27*:29–38, 1967.

O'Brien, T. F., del Pilar Pla, M., Mayer, K. H., *et al*. Intercontinental spread of a new antibiotic resistance gene on an epidemic plasmid. *Science 230*:87–88, 1985.

Roberts, M. C. Gene transfer in the urogenital and respiratory tract. In: *Gene Transfer in the Environment*, pp. 347–376. (Levy, S. B. and Miller, R. V. Eds.), McGraw-Hill, New York, 1989.

Rolland, R. M., Hausfater, G., Marshall, B., and Levy, S. B. Antibiotic-resistant bacteria in wild primates: Increased prevalence in baboons feeding on human refuse. *Appl. Env. Microbiol. 49*:791–794, 1985.

Sanders, C. C. New β-lactams: new problems for the internist. *Ann. Int. Med. 115*:650–651, 1991.

Smith, D. H. Salmonella with transferable drug resistance. *N. Engl. J. Med. 275*:625–630, 1966.

Sugarman, B. and Pesanti, E. Treatment failures secondary to *in vivo* development of drug resistance by microorganisms. *Rev. Infect. Dis. 2*:153–167, 1980.

Tauxe, R. V. Cavanagh, T. R. and Cohen, M. L. Interspecies gene transfer *in vivo* producing an outbreak of multiply resistant Shigellosis. *J. Infect. Dis. 160*:1067–1070, 1989.

Zscheck, K. K., Hull, R., and Murray, B. E. Restriction mapping and hybridization studies of a β-lactamase-encoding fragment from *Streptococcus* (*Enterococcus*) *faecalis*. *Antimicrob. Agents Chemother. 32*:768–769, 1988.

CHAPTER 5

Broome, C. V., Mortimer, E. A., Katz, S. L. *et al*. Use of chemoprophylaxis to prevent the spread of *Hemophilus influenzae* b in day-care facilities. *N. Engl. J. Med. 316*:1226–1228, 1987.

Classen, D. C. Evans, R. S., Pestotnik, S. L. *et al*. The timing of prophylactic administration of antibiotics and the risk of surgical-wound infection. *N. Engl. J. Med. 326*:281–286, 1992.

Col, N. F. and O'Connor, R. W. Estimating worldwide current antibiotic usage: Report of Task Force 1. *Rev. Infect. Dis. 9*:S232–243, 1987.

Knapp, J. S., Zenilman, J. M., Biddle, J. W. *et al*. Distribution and frequency of strains of *Neisseria gonorrhoeae* with plasmid-mediated, high-level resistance to tetracycline (TRNG) in the United States. *J. Infect. Dis. 155*:819–822, 1987.

Kunin, C. M., Lipton, H. L., Tupasi, T. *et al*. Social, behavioral and practical factors affecting antibiotic use worldwide: report of Task Force 4. *Rev. Infect. Dis. 9*:S270–285, 1987.

Morse, S. A. Antibiotic resistance in *Neisseria gonorrhoeae*: implications for future therapy. *APUA Newsletter 8*:4:1, 7–8, 1990.

Parker, C. W. Drug Allergy. *N. Engl. J. Med. 292*:732–736, 1975.

Reid, G. and Sobel, J. D. Bacterial adherence in the pathogenesis of urinary tract infection: a review. *Rev. Infect. Dis. 9*:470–487, 1987.

Seppala, H., Nissinen, A., Jarvinen, H. *et al.* Resistance to erythromycin in Group A streptococci. *N. Engl. J. Med. 326*:292–297, 1992.

Wald, E. R. Sinusitis in children. *N. Engl. J. Med. 326*:319–323, 1992.

CHAPTER 6

Anderson, E. S. and Lewis, M. J. Characterization of a transfer factor associated with drug resistance in *Salmonella typhimurium*. *Nature 208*:843–849, 1965.

Edel, W., Van Schothorsat, M., Van Leusden, F. M. and Kampelmacher, E.H. Epidemiological studies on *Salmonella* in a certain area. *Zbl. Bakt Hyg. I. Abt. Orig. A 242*:468–480, 1978.

Holmberg, S. D. *et al.* Drug resistant *Salmonella* from animals fed antibiotics. *N. Engl. J. Med. 311*:617–622, 1987.

Hummel, R., Tschape, H., and Witte, W. Spread of plasmid-mediated nourseothricin resistance in connection with antibiotic use in animal husbandry. *J. Basic Microb. 26*:461–466, 1986.

Levy, S. B. Antibiotic use for growth promotion in animals: ecologic and public health consequences. *J. Food Protection 50*:616–620, 1987.

Levy, S. B., Fitzgerald, G. G. and Macone, A. B. Changes in the intestinal flora of farm personnel after introduction of tetracycline-supplemented feed on a farm. *N. Engl. J. Med. 295*:583–588, 1976.

Lyons, R. W., Samples, C. L., DeSilva, H. N. *et al.* An epidemic of resistant *Salmonella* in a nursery: animal-to-animal spread. *J. Amer. Med. Assoc. 243*:546–547, 1980.

Marshall, B. M., Petrowski, D., and Levy, S. B. Inter and intraspecies spread of *E. coli* in a farm environment in the absence of antibiotic usage. *Proc. Nat'l Acad. Sci.* (USA) *87*:6609–6613, 1990.

Riley, L. W. *et al.* Evaluation of isolated cases of salmonellosis by plasmid profile analysis: introduction and transmission of a bacterial clone by precooked roast beef. *J. Infect. Dis. 148*:12–17, 1983.

Riley, L. W. *et al.* Importance of host factors in human salmonella caused by multiresistant strains of *Salmonella*. *J. Infect. Dis. 149*:878–883, 1984.

Ryan, C. A., Nickels, M. K. *et al.* Massive outbreak of antimicrobial-resistant salmonellosis traced to pasteurized milk. *J. Amer. Med. Assoc. 258*:3269–3279, 1987.

Schifferli, D. M. and Beachey, E. H. Bacterial adhesion: modulation by antibiotics which perturb protein synthesis. *Antimicrob. Agents Chemother. 32*:1603–1608, 1988.

Spika, J. S., Waterman, S. H., Soo Hoo, G. W. *et al.* Chloramphenicol-resistant *Salmonella newport* traced through hamburger to dairy farms. *N. Engl. J. Med.* *316*:565–580, 1987.

Stokstad, E. L. R. and Jukes, T. H. Further observations on the "animal protein factor." *Proc. Soc. Exp. Biol. Med. 73*:523–528, 1950.

CHAPTER 7

Agrios, G. N. *Plant Pathology*, 3rd edition. Academic Press, San Diego, pp. 510–608, 1988.

Ervin, M. A. Qualitative use assessment for streptomycin. Document 006306, Environmental Protection Agency, 1988.

Hirsh, D. C., Ling, G. V., and Ruby, A. L. Incidence of R-plasmids in fecal flora of healthy household dogs. *Antimicrob. Agents Chemother. 17*:313–315, 1980.

Levy, S. B. Antibiotic resistant bacteria in food of man and animals. In: *Antimicrobials and Agriculture* (Woodbine, M., Ed.). Butterworths, London, pp. 525–531, 1983.

Monaghan, C., Tierney, U., and Colleran, E. Antibiotic resistance and R-factors in the fecal coliform flora of urban and rural dogs. *Antimicrob. Agents Chemother. 19*:266–270, 1981.

Sundlof, S. F., Riviere, J. E. and Craigmill, A.L. *The Food Animal Residue Avoidance Databank Trade Name File*. Institute of Food and Agricultural Sciences, University of Florida, Gainesville, FL, 1989.

CHAPTER 8

Baquero, F., Martinez-Beltran, J., and Loza, E. A review of antibiotic resistance patterns of *Streptococcus pneumoniae* in Europe. *J. Antimicrob. Chemother. 28*: Suppl. C:31–38, 1991.

Bush, K. Excitement in the β-lactamase arena. *J. Antimicrob. Chemother. 24*:831–840, 1989.

Cruciani, R. A., Barker, J. L., Zasloff, M., Chen, H-C., and Colamonici, O. Antibiotic magainins exert cytolytic activity against transformed cell lines through channel formation. *Proc. Natl. Acad. Sci.* (USA) *88*:3792–3796, 1991.

Domenico, P., Hopkins, T., and Cunha, B. A. The effect of sodium salicylate on antibiotic susceptibility and synergy in *Klebsiella pneumoniae*. *J. Antimicrob. Chemother. 25*:343–351, 1990.

Gostin, L. O., Cleary, P.D., Mayer, K. H., Brandt, A. M., and Chittenden, E.H.

Screening immigrants and international travelers for the human immunodeficiency virus. *N. Engl. J. Med. 322*:1743–1746, 1990.

Kliebe C., Nies, B. A., Meyer, J. F. *et al.* Evolution of plasmid-coded resistance to broad-spectrum cephalosporins. *Antimicrob. Agents Chemother. 28*:302–307, 1985.

Lehrer, R. I. and Ganz, T. Antimicrobial polypeptides of human neutrophils. *Blood 76*:2169–2181, 1990.

Levy, S. B., and Novick, R. P. (Eds.) *Antibiotic Resistance Genes: Ecology, Transfer and Expression.* Cold Spring Harbor, NY, 1986.

Liss, R. H. and Batchelor, F. R. Economic evaluations of antibiotic use and resistance—a perspective report of Task Force 6. *Rev. Infect. Dis. 9*:S297–S312, 1987.

Skurray, R. A., Rouch, D. A., Lyon, B. R. *et al.* Multiresistant *Staphylococcus aureus*: genetics and evolution of epidemic Australian strains. *J. Antimicrob. Chemother. 21*: Suppl. C: 19–38, 1988.

Tuomanen, E. A single genetic locus on *Bordetella pertussis* controls virulence and tolerance to antibiotics. *APUA Newsletter 8*:4:5, 1990.

CHAPTER 10

Farrar, W. E., Jr. and Eidson, M. R factors in strains of *Shigella dysenteriae* type 1 isolated in the Western Hemisphere during 1969–1970. *J. Infect. Dis. 124*: 327–329.

Kunin, C. Problems in antibiotic usage. In: *Principles and Practice in Infectious Diseases*, 3rd Edition, (Mandel, G. L., Douglas, R. G. Jr., and Bennett, J. E., Eds.) Churchill Livingstone, New York, pp. 427–434, 1990.

Levy, S. B. Ecology of antibiotic resistance determinants. In: *Antibiotic Resistance Genes: Ecology, Transfer and Expression* (Levy, S. B., and Novick, R. P., Eds.), Cold Spring Harbor Press, New York, pp. 17–29, 1986.

Levy, S. B. Antibiotic availability and use: consequences to man and his environment. *J. Clin. Epidemiol. 44*:835–875, 1991.

Levy, S. B., Clowes, R. C., and Koenig, E. L. (Eds.), *Molecular Biology, Pathogenicity, and Ecology of Bacterial Plasmids.* Plenum Press, New York, 1981.

Liss, R. H. and Batchelor, F. R. Economic evaluations of antibiotic use and resistance—a perspective report of Task Force 6. *Rev. Infect. Dis. 9*:S297–S312, 1987.

Thamlikitkul, V. Antibiotic dispensing by drug store personnel in Bangkok, Thailand. *J. Antimicrob. Chemother. 21*:125, 1988.

INDEX